Contents

This book is dedicated
to
Dr Andrea Wild.

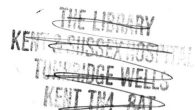

Primary Care in the Twenty-First Century

An international perspective

Geoff Meads

Professor of Organisational Research
Centre for Primary Health Care Studies
Warwick Medical School, University of Warwick

With country profiles prepared by Michiyo Iwami

Foreword by

Professor Yvonne Carter OBE, MD, FRCGP, FMedSci
Dean
Warwick Medical School, University of Warwick

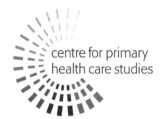

centre for primary
health care studies

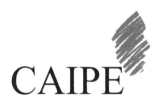

CAIPE

Radcliffe Publishing
Oxford • Seattle

Radcliffe Publishing Ltd
18 Marcham Road
Abingdon
Oxon OX14 1AA
United Kingdom

www.radcliffe-oxford.com
Electronic catalogue and worldwide online ordering facility.

British Library Cataloguing in Publication Data

A catalogue record for this book is available from the British Library

ISBN-10   1 85775 711 4
ISBN-13   978 1 85775 711 8

Typeset by Action Publishing Technology Ltd, Gloucester
Printed and bound by TJ International Ltd, Padstow, Cornwall

Foreword

I was honoured and delighted to receive an invitation from Professor Geoff Meads to write the Foreword to this book. Geoff is Professor of Organisational Research at the newly established Warwick Medical School at the University of Warwick. I have also worked with Geoff during his previous post at City University in London and in his leadership roles at the UK Centre for the Advancement of Interprofessional Education. He has written widely on international developments in health policy and public service relationships, and he is particularly well placed to guide the reader.

In the *Lancet* in 2004, Barbara Starfield wrote an article entitled: 'Is primary care essential?' She went on to write about how primary care is first contact, continuous, comprehensive and coordinated care for individuals and populations undifferentiated by age, gender, disease or organ system. As an academic discipline, primary care has achieved a remarkable position in the international healthcare scene during the past 50 years. It is still, however, widely regarded as a newcomer by many researchers from other disciplines, while those within it are seeing signs of a 'middle-age crisis'. This book explores how these two views can co-exist and is both timely and necessary.

Primary care, or its synonym family medicine, is a product of the 1950s: part of the fundamental re-evaluation of society that took place after the post-war generation challenged their surrounding world. In this era, the voice of the clinical generalist was heard as a reaction against the biomedical culture of the more traditional medical model in secondary or acute healthcare. These ideas shaped the development of one of the most fundamental concepts underpinning family practice: patient centredness.

Using in-depth case studies of individual countries, this book describes how family medicine is now practised within six forms of organisational development. Through examples of international collaboration, transferable learning between services and between professions in health and social care is strongly encouraged in order to promote the sharing of experiences as widely as possible. The importance of the parity of relationships is also clearly highlighted at the heart of health and social care.

This book is a welcome addition to the literature on international primary care. It illuminates the importance of comparative models in different healthcare systems and deals systematically with the subject. Understanding the issues that face primary care teams around the world is an important concept in preparing for future challenges, and this book clearly, concisely and very readably summarises the global story.

Professor Yvonne Carter OBE, MD, FRCGP, FMedSci
Dean
Warwick Medical School, University of Warwick
March 2006

Preface

The authoritative text on international primary care will have to wait. It will, almost certainly, not be written by the present author. What follows in this book is an academic and partial account, but also a personal one. For those interested, the research methodology is there to be scrutinised: a thematic analysis of case study data derived from semi-structured field interviews with purposive samples of 'leading edge' health policy makers and pioneer primary care practitioners across six continents, augmented by a systematic literature review and documentary searches.[1,2] But the application of the research methodology and its outcomes do not, of themselves, provide the material for this volume. Its findings are derived as much from the author's own previous experience of primary care as from the evidence garnered in studies of global developments during the 2002–2005 period. Previous roles, as primary care professional, manager, planner and policy maker, create the value base on which this book is founded.*

Such a base is, of course, actually a bias. We look in this book at contemporary primary care developments through the prism of relationships. Deliberately, our starting point is neither economic nor clinical, the two conventional perspectives, and the first the most common intellectual discipline for international health policy assessments.[3–5] Rather, our approach to primary care is guided by the conviction that its personalised public services remain critically significant to the social cohesion and social capital of every State because they are, at times of distress, disease and disadvantage, the extension of our families and closest friendships. As such, for each State, primary care relationships are important as a litmus test for public policy. They require constant and diligent political attention.

The way in which these relationships operate reflects a government's stewardship of its people. In consumerist times, when choice and competition are often popular prerequisites for effective local health services, the political challenge to government is considerable. In some countries of Central Asia and Central America, for example, it may even amount to the issue on which the restoration and maintenance of civil society depends. Globally, there are still many echoes here of nineteenth-century Germany and Great Britain. In these two countries, individual primary care professions and businesses have their roots in government policies for the poor and their elevation into a fit enough labour (or fighting) force for the purposes of the Industrial Revolution (or war). In the post-millennium period, contemporary primary care development may actually still be as paternalistic, with undercurrents of social compliance, vested

---

* The author was a regional NHS director for primary care and performance management prior to his academic appointments. He is a qualified social worker and has advised the Department of Health, the Cabinet Office and several foreign governments on health policy issues during the period of the present international research programme.

interests, central elitism and political control; but increasingly too its organisational changes are pivotal features of participatory democracy in its many different, emerging forms.

In the pages that follow the focus will often be on these forms and the impact of 'modernisation', but the framework for the analysis will still be that of primary care's traditional key relationships:

- longitudinal comprehensive care for the individual
- the harnessing of resources in the family network and its context
- mobilising sources of community support
- advocacy both for and against government as the personal and particular circumstances require.

In short, we are interested in the ethics as much as the economics of primary care in the twenty-first century. While at the dawn of the new millennium the latter may seem prevalent in policy makers' decision making, primary care development remains, in practice, always a negotiation between central and local forces. Its encounters are *per se* micro-political events, unique separate transactions, each adding to accumulated and changing patterns of relationships in primary care. In these, ethical issues are paramount still. Moral as much as financial value must underpin modern primary care and its future direction.

The preparation of this volume owes much to many who share this conviction. Not least among these are Barbara Clague, Helena Low, Helen Betts and those at the UK Centre for the Advancement of Interprofessional Education. Their endorsement for the book is much appreciated. My colleagues in the International Primary Care (IPC) Unit at the Centre for Primary Health Care Studies, led by Professor Jeremy Dale in the University of Warwick, over the past three years have been an invaluable support. Dr Frances Griffiths, Patrick Wakida, Helen Tucker, Dr Maria Stuttaford, Dr Andrea Wild and, especially for this book, Michiyo Iwami have been those who have joined me in specific site visits and national case studies. Michiyo has drawn on these to compile a comprehensive international database of post-2000 primary care developments, which she used in drafting the individual country profiles that are regular inserts in the pages that follow. Michiyo herself has been a doctoral student throughout the period of the IPC Unit's programme, undertaking in parallel an in-depth investigation of women's health issues in Peru, and our hope is that this book will be of use not just to those engaged in primary care activities but also to those following in her footsteps as trainee researchers and postgraduate scholars. Both Michiyo and I would like to express our gratitude to Catherine Beckett, our assistant who has, with painstaking care, helped prepare our manuscript.

Much of our writing, literary and documentary research has taken place at the British Library, the Office for National Statistics, the University of Winchester and the King's Fund in London. We would also like to thank the staff of all four for their support and helpfulness.

Colleagues from other countries who have contributed to the information and ideas contained in this text are so many that it seems almost invidious to name specific individuals. Inevitably there will be many unfortunate and accidental omissions. But nevertheless, it would feel wrong not to acknowledge explicitly at least some of those who have helped us so much, with several staff from British embassies and Councils around the world deserving a special mention. Just as it was a surprise at the end of our study to find that primary care in the United Kingdom, for all its flaws and loose ends, compared so well with all the other models we encountered abroad, so too was it an unexpected pleasure to find our overseas representatives so unfailingly resourceful in locating the right people in the right places at the right times on our behalf.

So simply, by country in alphabetical order, and with an arbitrary limit of two per State, Michiyo and I would like to express our appreciation to the following individuals and all their colleagues:

Jane Conway (Australia)
Dr Dimitri Pond (Australia)
Dr Silvia Salinas (Bolivia)
Sara Shields (Bolivia)
Dr Joceline Oliveira (Brazil)
Rosalina Batista (Brazil)
Alan Richmond (Canada)
Micheline Nimmock (Canada)
Maria Pia Gazzella (Chile)
Dr Rodrigo Soto (Chile)
Zhang Zhong Jiu (China)
Dr Sijuan Fu (China)
Michael Valdes-Scott (Colombia)
Dr Julio Ospina (Colombia)
Marielos Benevides (Costa Rica)
Dr Luis Meneses (Costa Rica)
Dr Alena Petrakova (Czech Republic)
Dr Jan Holcick (Czech Republic)
Victoria Harrison (Finland)
Professor Pertti Kekki (Finland)
Dr Mamas Theodorou (Greece)
Dr Christos Leonis (Greece)
Dr Jeremy Shiffman (Indonesia)
Surayati Tucker (Indonesia)
Dr Tomonori Izawa (Japan)
Dr Kei Miyoshi (Japan)

Dr Luis Duran (Mexico)
Louise Batcheldor (Mexico)
Professor Lawrence Malcolm (New Zealand)
Robert Sloane (New Zealand)
Dr Ariel Frisancho (Peru)
Dr Juan Arroyo Laguna (Peru)
Mylene Beltran (Philippines)
Dr Elizabeth Paterno (Philippines)
Dr Paula Santana (Portugal)
Dr Antonio Rodrigues (Portugal)
Rev Mark Poh (Singapore)
Dr Eric Chian (Singapore)
Dr David Cameron (South Africa)
Dr Ivan Toms (South Africa)
Dr Visal Yawaponsiri (Thailand)
Chutatip Siripak (Thailand)
Dr Jonathan Gaifuba (Uganda)
Dr Nelson Sewankambo (Uganda)
Pippa Bagnall (UK)
Dr Sheila Adam (UK)
Dr Gregorio Sanchez (Venezuela)
Dr Miguel Angel de Lima (Venezuela)
Dr Orvill Adams (WHO)
Dr Rafael Bengoa (WHO)

A concluding note of gratitude must go to our partners, Patricia and Michael de Tisi, who have had to endure too many both physical and emotional absences because of this book and its preparation. I promise this is the last. Until the next time. And the final word must be for Dr Yvonne Carter, a general medical practitioner herself and Dean of the new Warwick Medical School. She it was, back in London in 2000, who provided the essential encouragement for the idea of such an international research programme and publication when, in most people's eyes, it was no more than yet another of the author's irrelevant eccentricities.

Geoff Meads
March 2006

References

1 Meads G, Iwami M, Wild A (2005) Transferable learning from international primary care developments. *International Journal of Health Planning and Management.* **20**: 253–67.

2 Meads G, Iwami M (2005) Health systems and development. In: Huque A, Zafarullah H (eds) *International Development and Governance*, pp. 803–20. New York: Taylor and Francis LLC.

3 Flood C (2000) *International Health Care Reform. A legal, economic and political analysis.* London: Routledge.

4 Lassey M, Lassey W, Jinks M (1997) *Health Care Systems Around The World: characteristics, issues, reforms.* New Jersey: Prentice Hall.

5 Perkins B (1999) Re-forming medical delivery systems: economic organisation and dynamics of regional planning and managed competition. *Social Science and Medicine.* **48**: 241–51.

Chapter I

International approach

Terms of reference

Thirty-three countries and 34 months. Democracies only; with the possible exception of Cuba, given its sustained global influence over the organisation of primary care. Dr Che Guevara and President Fidel Castro as the founding fathers of Health for All policies: if they shaped international developments during the second half of the twentieth century who are the formative forces for the first half of the present one? Such a fundamental question needs a clear and cogent analysis: robust terms of reference are required.

So, back to our defining agenda. Only countries with major health policy reforms over the past decade, and preferably since 1997 when the New Labour Government came into power in the United Kingdom. Even better if the changes are post-millennium and parallel Prime Minister Tony Blair's mantra of 'Modernisation' for a 'New NHS'. Fortunately the organisational developments of many countries more or less do.

And, for the purposes of comparability, small countries are mostly ruled out. Take ten million as the arbitrary minimum population. But again, on the advice of two directors of the World Health Organization (WHO), there need to be exceptions to the general rule. Some countries are in effect experimental laboratories for modernising and primary care-based health policies – Uganda, Kyrgyzstan and Georgia for instance are, we learnt, sometimes seen informally by global policy makers as three such action research sites. Others ape the complexity of political process and decision making found in larger nation states; and worldwide devolutionary pressures mean, perhaps, that some provinces might even be considered. Ontario (Canada), Oaxaco (Mexico), New South Wales (Australia), Lara (Venezuela) and Northern Ireland, for example, come to mind; but probably not in their own right. Ultimately they are illustrations of the new extended limits of national health policies for local resource management. But, of course, small country success stories should at least be mentioned, where they fit the criteria. Costa Rica and New Zealand definitely, Singapore too, and Greece simply because it seems to be experimenting with the introduction of every health policy reform yet invented; and simultaneously.

So, back to the criteria again. We are looking to make sense of primary care in the twenty-first century. Our perspective is global and our lens alights on developments in countries with novel organisational formations in primary care. These developments have broadly common characteristics. They are partnership based and public health oriented. Their new collaborative approaches to the wider local control of health services and resources require new forms of governance and regulation. Usually these primary care organisations are not only interprofessional in their practice but intersectoral in their management.

Non-governmental public action is a critical component. Communities play a larger part in the executive functions than previously, but in very different ways in very different places: a spectrum stretching from commercial to charitable representation. And, on all fronts, these organisational developments are more open to international influences, through globalisation, than ever before. We live, as the Chinese say, in interesting times and, of course, China itself as the world's largest country, its 'Middle Kingdom', must be included.

Making sense of such times, through defining their direction of travel, is our task in this book. Its preparation has itself involved much travel: 75 flights in one year alone, 280 000 kilometres in all. Along the way more than 200 interviews and 50 visits to local primary care organisations: each one identified by a 'lead' national policy maker as an exemplar of future practice developments. In total, an exhilarating experience and an educational one, leading to numerous follow-up exchanges, both personal and academic, and a plethora of joint articles, shared ideas and curricula, and proposals for further research collaborations.* The theme has been 'transferable learning', with common policy principles the framework for adaptation if not adoption of one site's programmes by its prospective partners elsewhere.[1]

As terms of reference, all the above parameters seem to have come together to produce a successful product. A one-year project became a proposed seven-year-long research unit (to 2008). For the author, one fellowship led to another, and NHS grant funding throughout 2002–05 was annually renewed with 'strong' ratings from reviewers. Published articles total more than 20 and this is already the second book, augmenting a series of chapters in other volumes, with some even attracting overseas translations into other languages.[2–5] There seems to be a thirst for new knowledge through the kinds of multinational exchanges and communications now possible, while just within policy circles of the UK the emphasis on 'joined-up government' has meant briefings and seminars not only at the Strategy Unit of the Ministry of Health but also in the Home Office, the Treasury and, inevitably, the Cabinet Office itself.

As time has passed so such inputs have increasingly, and not infrequently, been requested elsewhere: for example, from the Midland Health Services Executive in Eire; from the major national health insurance corporation in Mexico (IMSS); from the global organisation for the promotion of community-based healthcare education at its 2003 and 2005 annual conferences in Australia and Vietnam (Network-TUFH); from the Inter-Americas Social Security Association in the Dominican Republic; and finally, from the individuals at WHO (Geneva) itself. The level of demand corresponds to the level of dilemma about the future of primary care and its organisation. In terms of growth, the twentieth century belonged essentially to family medicine and its practice. The twenty-first century clearly does not. In the 1990s in England, it was still quite possible for a leading British professional commentator to write, with minimal challenge, that primary care and general practice were synonymous.[6] The name of the service was also that of the profession, the surgery and

---

* The research has been reported regularly in a series of 2003–2005 articles for Medicom's *Primary Care Report*, which has been the most-read journal in NHS primary care trusts in England.

the vocational training course. Ten years later it was all change. In just one decade, official documents in the UK relegated the general practitioner (GP) to seventh in the pecking order for direct patient access: behind the triage nurse and community pharmacist, walk-in and healthy living centres, and, of course, the online information and telephone advice services of NHS Direct.[7] Moreover, this list does not include, because it pre-dates it, the subsequent drive for more self-managed care, backed up by better educational inputs and preventive measures (e.g. on diet, exercise, birth control) from non-NHS agencies.

As the service profile of primary care diversified so its structures and processes have had to change. It is now, by definition, a complex organisation. The simple forms of hierarchic bureaucracy or peer-based partnerships are inadequate, seem to be rapidly passing away and can no longer apply to future developments. At least not as the main organisational vehicles, unlike in the past. Historic strengths should endure, be protected even, but conservatism clearly has its constraints in terms of understanding the future agencies of and for primary care: in terms of their accountabilities, management, operational mechanisms, investment profiles and human resources; and indeed even their ownership. Constructive scenario planning rather than single strategies is needed to take primary care forward, given its new range of different constituents. The international overview provides a rich resource for mapping the alternative routes to 2100. If it is true that primary care must always be locally negotiated, it is also now the case that its future depends as much on international policy and practice influences as it ever did in the past on professional self-determination. If this is the conclusion reached by researchers in such countries as Zambia,[8] Colombia and Mozambique,[9] how much more applicable may it be to the larger, more economically developed and therefore more interdependent States of Western Europe and North America?

The cast list

The 24 countries that have been the subject of specific studies can be divided into four groups. Together they supply most of the material for this book. Not enough clearly, but rather more than some previous texts, which have asserted global 'truths' on the basis of evidence derived from as few as four to six countries.[10,11] Our research framework, in geographic terms, does at least cover all the main continents, although North Africa, the Middle East and the Indian subcontinent are conspicuous by their absence, except as literature references. This omission arises largely from the democratic deficit of recent 'modernising' reforms in many of the States of these regions, plus a shortfall in reliable research. Our framework, too, also covers the six discernible models of mainstream primary care organisation that we define and explain in Chapter 2, and then illustrate in detail in the narrative of the rest of this book. Based on the terms of reference set out above, the research framework facilitated our deliberations as we arrived at the following focus for our fieldwork.

The first cluster of countries identified for study were those which scored on each of the five criteria or dimensions of modernisation we identified at the outset, through our meetings with NHS policy makers and our reviews of their principal academic sources in terms of policy theorists and commentators.[12,13]

Accordingly, in each national health system there was first a contemporary reform process under way promoting a form of local resource management in primary care. This process also included, second, new collaborations across the public and independent sectors, and third, attempts at more significant community participation. In every setting, the emergent organisations have been subject to, fourth, new forms of regulation as governments seek to exercise effectively their national stewardship roles in public health. And fifth and finally, in all of the following 12 countries we found examples, from our literature searches and documentary reviews, of innovations in the area of interprofessional learning and development. Several of these have now been published.[14]

Together these five criteria represent the dimensions of a partnership-based health system founded on modern primary care organisations. Our first cluster of countries for fieldwork enquiry in 2003–04 comprised:

- Canada
- Chile
- Finland
- Greece
- Japan
- New Zealand
- Peru
- Philippines
- Portugal
- South Africa
- Thailand
- Uganda

plus, of course, England and, as our pilot site from a preliminary research visit in 2001, Brazil.

In 2003, we returned to Rio de Janeiro for a short follow-up study. By this time the interest in and the financial support for our programme had grown to the extent that we were able to incorporate into our standard fieldwork approach the countries placed on our reserve list. In each of these, at least one of the main dimensions of modernisation was missing, but equally, on one of the other dimensions, there were indications of developments that might be of particular value in terms of international transferable learning. The 'Big Bang' change management style of Bogotá's decentralisation and the 'experimental' values-based orientation of new medical and healthcare curricula designs in New South Wales were two such examples of this potential. The full list comprised:

- Australia
- Bolivia
- China
- Colombia
- Costa Rica
- Czech Republic
- Indonesia
- Mexico

- Singapore
- Venezuela.

The writer and his team undertook fieldwork in all of the above countries in 2004/05. In each, a minimum of two national policy leaders and two local representatives of exemplar organisational developments in primary care were normally the subjects of semi-structured interviews using the same topic guide for transferable learning. In many cases, further interviews were arranged, at the invitation of our various hosts, to provide supplementary information and intelligence. The volume of interviews and visits could reach to a dozen, in a single country.

For our last group of countries a rationale such as that outlined above, with its rational selection process, cannot be claimed. They, in effect, chose themselves. If it was not quite outright opportunism, the motif for research in the following sites does come down to individual interests and associations: sometimes based on the past and personal links of members of the Warwick University IPC research group (as, for instance, in the case of Turkey) and sometimes through invitations from local sites seeking to be included in a new international research project (as, for example, in the case of the Rhondda health services in Wales looking to initiate 'Active User and Carer Involvement' programmes). There were nine countries in the last, very disparate cluster. They are as follows:

- Croatia
- Dominican Republic
- Ireland
- Kenya
- Scotland
- Slovenia
- Spain
- Turkey
- Wales.

Visits to the above were scattered across the 2002–05 time frame for the research programme, with data collected on an *ad hoc* basis around attendance at meetings, workshops and conferences. As sources, this cluster is best thought of as merely providing background intelligence. While some of the opportunistic research on, for example, developments in community-based medical education (in Eldoret, Kenya) has been reported elsewhere,[15] none of the detailed case accounts of Chapters 3 to 8 is derived from this grouping. No more are any universal assertions. Neither the information this research supplied nor the techniques employed in the data acquisition would properly sustain generalisable case studies.

The 33 countries above are our cast list. The United States of America is not included but, as we will see, the American influence is still everywhere and its own developments are often the starting point for both action and analysis, either tacitly or explicitly,[16,17] in much of recent international health systems comparative research. But for our purposes, in terms of relationship-based primary care and organisational developments which accord with our five key collaborative criteria of modernisation, the USA does not fit. As a result, the door is open for a wider international exchange, especially between developing and developed countries. It is, I think, an unusual but attractive prospect.

Supporting acts

It is also a proposition now firmly supported by the WHO. Particularly in the early design stages of our programme, WHO staff could not have been more helpful. The phone call from one of its senior members, who was attending a meeting in the Balkans, to check that I was being looked after and could find the data I was seeking on my first visit to his Swiss office still sticks in the memory. Apart from being a singular act of long-distance kindness, it brought home to me the inter-connectedness now of contemporary developments and the feasibility of seeing these truly through a worldwide perspective.

At the Geneva WHO headquarters the global perspective in the post-millennium period is changing subtly. Poverty is replacing primary healthcare *per se* as the principal priority for those addressing the public health improvement agenda. Sustainable development is their touchstone.[18] This is a logical progression on past policies, which represents more than just a change in the top-table leadership of the WHO. The 1978 Alma Ata principles were officially reaffirmed at WHO-sponsored events in 1998, but after more than 20 years there has been a sense not only of fatigue but also of frustration in that so many of the Health for All targets have either been underachieved or sidelined. The focus on mainstream poverty since the WHO Annual Report of 2000 has sought to counter diversionary tactics, especially in dictatorships and some consumerist Western countries, by taking the Alma Ata 'Pillar' principles[19] of cross-boundary collaboration and community participation and extending them beyond the traditional limits of healthcare provision to the full range of public service delivery sectors, in pursuit of enhanced social and economic status for entire populations.

In Europe, this has meant using a range of economic and employment levers to promote an international labour market in healthcare professionals and to stimulate across the continent new waves of social and ambulatory care providers in the independent sector. Long-term European shortfalls in terms of nursing supply and response to special needs and migrant minorities are being addressed,[20] and in each country the profile of primary care is becoming more diverse and differentiated as a result.

In the UK in particular, the post-2000 NHS 'journey for major improvement' is being routed through 'a much wider choice of different types of health services' characterised at the frontline by more 'personalised' and 'faster treatment'. For primary care this is said to mean 'new ways of meeting patients' needs', 'new flexibilities', 'a wider range of providers including independent sector organisations' and 'an enhanced range and quality of services'.[21] For the Ministry itself the first policy task is a new White Paper on 'out-of-hospital care' and the first 'distinctive' role for the Department of Health in 'developing strategy and direction for the health and social care system' is to 'include not-for-profit and private providers – while maintaining (of course) the integrity of the system and its values'.[22]

The message could not be clearer. The local contracts and quality initiatives of the personal medical services and practice-based commissioning programmes were not ends in themselves. Further organisational developments are anticipated. As with education, social care and social housing, these are expected to embrace non-professionals and new participants. Our interviews with NHS senior and middle managers around the UK over the period 2003–05 indicated that, on the ground, they clearly recognised the real underlying direction of travel. The following are typical of their questions, the responses to which we have reported elsewhere.[23,24]

- How can tomorrow's primary care organisations achieve a parity of interests between their different stakeholders?
- Can new primary care and non-governmental organisations combine to extend primary care and public participation?
- What works and where? (And how do we learn about it?)
- Is it possible to get primary care professionals 'onside' with modern policies?
- Will the new organisational developments release more potential for primary care?
- What will be the impact on public accountability (and personal trust) of more diversity and choice?

All of the above are wrapped up in the simplest and most frequently asked question: 'What should be the defining characteristics of modern primary care organisations?' This is the question that this book addresses. In the UK, it is impossible to do so without first reflecting on the future role of the GP. In the next chapter, employing our international perspective, this is where we start.

References

1 Meads G, Iwami M, Wild A (2005) Transferable learning from international primary care developments. *International Journal of Health Planning and Management*. **20**: 253–67.
2 Meads G, Ashcroft J, Barr H et al. (2005) *The Case for Interprofessional Collaboration: in health and social care*. Oxford: Blackwell Science.
3 Meads G, Griffiths F, Iwami M et al. (2005) Lecciones Internacionales para Nuevas Prácticas Organizacionales en la Atención Primaria. *Revista Seguridad Social*. **252**: 1–12.
4 Meads G, Iwami M (2005) Health systems and development. In: Huque A, Zafarullah (eds) *International Development Governance*, pp. 803–20. New York: Taylor and Francis LLC.
5 Meads G (2005) Family medicine: future issues and perspectives. In: García-Peña C, Muñoz O, Duran L et al. (eds) *Family Medicine at the Dawn of the 21st Century*, pp.17–33. Mexico City: Instituto Mexicano de Seguro Social.
6 Pereira Gray D (1995) Primary care and public health. *Health and Hygiene*. **16**: 49–62.
7 Department of Health (2004) *A Responsive and High-quality Local NHS*. London: DoH.
8 Hearst N, Blas E (2001) Learning from experience: research on health sector reform in the developing world. *Health Policy Plan*. **16** (supplement): 1–3.
9 Pfeiffer J (2003) International NGOs and primary health care in Mozambique. *Social Science and Medicine*. **56**: 725–38.
10 Powell F, Wessen A (eds) (1999) *Health Care Systems in Transition*. London: Sage.
11 Mullan F (1998) The 'Mona Lisa' of health policy: primary care at home and abroad. *Health Affairs*. **17**: 118–26.

12 Coote A, Hunter D (1996) *New Agenda for Health*. London: Institute for Public Policy Research.

13 Giddens A (1998) *The Third Way. The Renewal of Social Democracy*. London: Polity Press.

14 Wild A, Meads G (2005) Practice teaching in a global world. *Journal of Practice Teaching*. **5**(3): 5–19.

15 Wild A, Meads G (2006) Practice learning in a global world. In: Ixer G (ed.) *Practice Learning: perspectives on globalisation, citizenship and cultural change*. London: Whiting and Birch.

16 Perkins B (1999) Re-forming medical delivery systems: economic organisation and dynamics of regional planning and managed competition. *Social Science and Medicine*. **48**: 241–51.

17 World Bank (1993) *Investing in Health*. Washington, DC: World Bank.

18 Fransen L (2001) Partners in health and poverty. *Development*. **44**(1): 129–31.

19 Macdonald J (1992) *Primary Health Care. Medicine in its place*. London: Earthscan.

20 Ludvigsen C, Roberts K (1996) *Health Care Policies and Europe*. London: Butterworth-Heinemann.

21 Department of Health (2004) *The NHS Improvement Plan. Putting people at the heart of services*. London: DoH.

22 Department of Health (2005) *Forward Plan 2005–2006*. London: DoH.

23 Wild A, Iwami M, Meads G (2003) Different systems, same issues. *Primary Care Report*. **5**(16): 14–19.

24 Meads G, Wild A, Griffiths F et al. (2006) The management of new primary care organisations: an international perspective. *Health Services Management Research*. **11**(2): 1–8.

Chapter 2

Future options for family medicine

Introduction

It is ten years since I first visited the subject of this chapter in print under nigh on the same title, again at the invitation of the present publisher.* Then, my perspective was determined exclusively by events and experience in the UK. The theme of the book was that the lead primary care professionals in the NHS were in an unprecedented position to create and control the direction of health services, through an exciting range of organisational developments that combined providing and purchasing roles. Now, from an international perspective, the toughest truth for many practitioners of family medicine** is that its future is not in their own hands. The principle of professional self-determination is no longer sufficient or even sometimes regarded as relevant in the expanding practice of modern primary care services. The investment and consequent accountabilities these require stretch far beyond the regulatory rights of Royal Colleges or other exclusive unidisciplinary forms of protective professional association for family medicine.

Autonomy has become a relational concept, earnt in everyday practice by family doctors through effective collaboration with other practitioners, the public and their patients, as well as new partner agencies and policy makers. Personal trust and status for the general medical practitioner cannot be taken for granted. Family medicine itself as a clinical code of conduct may essentially, over time, stay the same, but its organisational behaviour, even in the medium term, cannot but change with the emergent post-millennium political contexts. The future of the general medical practitioner, as a result, can be viewed as largely an external rather than an internal issue, and as such an international perspective may provide at least as helpful a position from which to appreciate future options as the narrower British standpoint did a decade ago.

* The edited book was entitled *Future Options for General Practice* and was published in 1996 by the then Radcliffe Medical Press (Oxford). Its contributors, almost all of whom were British general medical practitioners, set out ten alternative organisational models for primary care. Some of these have disappeared without trace, but others proved remarkably robust, including the first proposal for an NHS primary care trust.

** This chapter focuses on the medical practitioner in general practice, the most significant single player historically in primary care. As general practice is a term now often used loosely to cover other personnel as well, in this chapter to avoid confusion the term 'family medicine' is used, while acknowledging that in many places 'family medicine' and 'general medical practice' do constitute different grades and even philosophies of clinical care.

Organisational context

In global terms, family medicine is now practised within six forms of organisational development. In this chapter I will look to explore the different and defining features of each of these, presenting them conceptually as 'ideal types' and empirically as aggregates of cited local examples from both our research and the relevant literature across broad-based, continental-scale geographic areas. The impact of cultural conditioning will be clear, but so too will be the consistent and powerful political motif of multinational modernisation. Globally, family medicine cannot escape its transformational tendencies. For example, however distinctive particular approaches to local resource management may be, universally the decentralisation of health systems requires family medicine to assume new executive and educational roles.[1] Its historic roots in poverty are undermined by new policies and professions that espouse the poor and promote public health as paths to their own preservation and progress. Not infrequently the family doctor is left virtually friendless by modern organisational developments in primary care. The paternal and sometimes paternalistic relationship with nurses is a thing of the past: they have often become graduates themselves, with their own prescribing rights and professional bodies. Personal administrators have been replaced by general management, and extended primary care means an emphasis on new community-based specialisms, often as alternatives to family medicine. These are now bidding, sometimes successfully, to substitute for some of its former functions. And, moreover, they are doing so at a lower cost in new and alternative settings, frequently with other organisations of either their own or their 'stakeholders' design. For the latter, they represent tomorrow's world of partnerships, public health improvement, popular trust and, not least, potential profit.

As a result, family medicine is no longer a discrete enterprise. It flourishes most where it has effective political alliances. These may sometimes, as in Moldova and Latvia for example, be with international and charitable sponsors,[2] or as in Estonia through government subsidy,[3] but they are rarely with other doctors. Or with the wealthy. Growth in medical specialisms and popular prosperity both threaten the foundations of the family doctor, as can their own pursuit of affluence. Across the world there are examples of family medicine becoming too expensive: pricing itself out of popular primary care development as, for instance, has recently happened in both Croatia and South Africa. Traditionally, partnership has been an important value for family medicine. It has often meant close and even commercial relationships between GPs. For the future of family medicine, and its maintenance, it will need to mean more outward-facing and less self-interested relationships. In Australia, the Commonwealth set out a series of critical stakeholders for the future in its review of 'General practice changing the future through partnerships'.[4] This new relational emphasis is apparent as we turn now to our classification of modern organisational developments in primary care.

Organisational developments

The six models or ideal types are as follows.

Extended general practice

Still dominant in much of Western Europe and, through past colonial influences, in countries such as those of the Caribbean, where British (and Spanish) political and cultural structures, in particular, have been adopted, the extended general practice remains one of the two basic global reference points for the development and practice of family medicine. Its counterpart is the district health system, which we describe below, and each possesses in the WHO and WONCA (World Organization of National Colleges and Academies of General Practice) an overarching and powerful sponsor with widespread international influence.

Although the extended general practice has emerged from the individualistic and sometimes idiosyncratic practice of independent medical professionals, it is now firmly team based with a multiprofessional profile. Nevertheless, family medicine is its pivotal and principal source of interventions. These interventions may include, increasingly, chronic disease management and some clinical prevention procedures, but they remain focused on diagnosing and treating the individual patient who is offered personal care with a named doctor through a registered list. Values of continuity, trust and reciprocity apply in what is a holistic approach to family medicine. In the modern extended general practice, this approach legitimises the role of the family doctor as not just the referral point but also the gatekeeper for secondary and sometimes social care.

But the legitimacy now is only viable because it embraces others alongside the family doctor. Such are the contemporary and future pressures on scarce secondary and social care resources that an appeal simply to the traditional ethics and philosophies of general medical practice is never going to be enough. Family medicine needs new allies even within its most established stronghold of the GP surgery. Here its new partners are usually primary care nurses and managers, both growing in number and scope, plus several allied health professionals attracted by the ready prospect of increased resources, referrals, specialist roles and subsequent status. Counsellors, physiotherapists and dispensers are the most evident in this category, and while the doctor remains not only the lead partner and team leader, the practice and ownership of family medicine in the extended general practice is increasingly shared. Primary care nurse-led triage, prescribing and screening programmes are the most obvious examples of this change, which also applies, although to a lesser extent, to others in the developing primary care teams. GP-supervised (if only nominally) back pain programmes by practice-based physiotherapists are one common illustration of the latter and there are many others emerging, especially as long-stay institutional closures lead to a growing range of mental health issues for family medicine to address.

These issues have led in such countries as Sweden, Finland and England, where the extended general practice is in its most advanced form, to the transfer of major financial resource management responsibilities to representatives of family medicine from both local and national governments (e.g. NHS primary care trusts and individual or multi-practice-based commissioning in England). Incorporated within these transfers is an extended pastoral role in relation to conditions previously beyond the defined limits of medicine, and to the consequent inclusion in the practice unit of social workers and social care assistants. In poorer countries, like Barbados or Estonia, where through the British or Scandinavian influence the extended general practice is also being promoted as the main source of comprehensive longitudinal healthcare, such new roles may be undertaken by paid volunteers or part-time personnel. They signal the new proactive character of family medicine within the extended general practice. Although still essentially site based and demand driven, it does, in the twenty-first century, recognise its patients collectively as well as individually. They in return perceive their family doctor not simply as a personal physician and independent practitioner, but as the lead local healthcare professional whose growing team status is now very much *primus inter pares*.[5]

Managed care enterprise

Where the extended general practice is still a small (but growing) business, often with strong family and historic roots, the managed care enterprise is a recent phenomenon and novel form of corporate development. As such it is a modern, complex type of organisation in its collaborative structures and external stakeholder interactions, which eschews the simple hierarchic and peer partnership processes that have always applied in the past to general medical practice. For the family doctor in the managed care enterprise protocol, procedure and payment underpin clinical behaviour. While originally drawing on much of the GP gatekeeping experience and looking prospectively to incorporate extended general practices within its parameters, the managed care enterprise is essentially a product with a premium, where general management and the market, rather than the individual profession or patient, set the strategic direction. The managed care enterprise, of course, comes ultimately from the US and the commercial insurance industry.

Although it remains a minority organisational unit for family medicine globally, the managed care enterprise is growing and it is now the most frequently cited development in the relevant contemporary research literature (see, for example, Cabiedes and Guillen[6] and Flood[7]). Inevitably, by both design and default, the US influence is immensely powerful internationally, not least through its major donor charities and its leading financial and political contributions to the World Bank. As a result, the managed care enterprise is now turning up in unexpected locations. It is perhaps no surprise to see its establishment in the merged public-private Sickness Funds of Israel, Germany and the Netherlands, or in the care packages offered by the family health networks of Canada and Mexico, just across the borders from the US. But it is a surprise, perhaps even a shock, to discover similar programmes emerging over the past decade in, for example, Sri Lanka (under strong World Bank influence), Central Peru (with consultancy from Johns Hopkins University in Baltimore) and, almost incredibly given some of their past quasi-communist political positions, in articles reviewing developments in impoverished Zambia, Nigeria and Tanzania (each of which has been subject to International Monetary Fund conditions for mixed public-private service development in return for loan support and debt relief).[8-10]

The managed care enterprise is centrally characterised by the purchasing of family medicine as cost- and clinically effective supply side provision. When converted into a formal knowledge management process, through the systematic application of current information technologies and scientifically sound evidence, this purchasing activity becomes commissioning. It moves from a relationship of supply and demand to one of defined needs and resources as currencies, with both health and economic outputs as outcomes. The managed care enterprise is viewed by its architects as an integral part of a dynamic transactional market in which the general medical practitioner can occupy a series of roles as care manager, commodity broker and even payer. In this context, the family doctor is less expensive than other specialisms of medicine. The role is also more malleable. It acquires, as a result, different nomenclatures in a diversity or choice of providers, as the managed care enterprise looks to constrain hospital costs, maximise the value of its own frontline services and, through regular market research, reprofile demand in the interests of its own income and areas of expertise. In this context, family doctors may be termed, for example, 'general practitioners with special interest' (by English primary care trusts) or 'community GP specialists' (by German health insurance corporations). They are able to work, for instance, in 'point of service networks' (in New Zealand's Independent Practice Associations), supplying 'packages of care' everywhere and usually within the terms of the US-style 'programme budgets' originally drawn up by health maintenance organisations in California, Boston and Minneapolis.

Where the extended general practice is professionally oriented in its approach to family medicine, the managed care enterprise is firmly functional. The former will still lay claim to a normative commitment from its participants. In the managed care enterprise this commitment is unequivocally calculative. As such, it is at least as much an economic as social policy development. In those countries that are its leading exponents, issues surrounding the future of family medicine belong politically as much to Finance, Employment and Interior Ministries as they do to central Departments of Health. Recent attempts to privatise primary care in Portugal and extend family medicine coverage through government-supported independent health insurance agencies (ISAPREs) in Chile are two ready illustrations.[11,12] That neither were particularly effective indicates, contrary to what is often supposed, that the managed care enterprise may be growing internationally but this does not mean it will automatically become the prevalent framework globally for practitioners of family medicine.

Reformed polyclinic

Contrary to a popular opinion the polyclinic does not seem destined merely for extinction. It has not disappeared with the demise of the old Soviet Union. Indeed it is alive and kicking, and in unexpected places, not just Eastern Europe, and with a fresh *raison d'être*.

This rationale is not simply as a vehicle for privatisation, although in countries such as Hungary, and Russia itself in the early 1990s, polyclinic doctors were certainly in the vanguard of the shift to capitalism. Sometimes, in the absence of effective regulation, this was with disastrous consequences. By 1994, for example, the City Council of Riga, the capital of Latvia, found itself drastically downgrading medical fee scales during a period of consultancy by the author, as up to 60 specialists in a single polyclinic sought to expand both their roles and their remuneration by simply increasing referrals to each other of the same patients within their clinic. Payment was, in those days, based entirely on the number of consultations: each contact attracting a further fee for service.

Fortunately in Latvia, as elsewhere, matters have moved on. Russian medical schools had already pioneered the inclusion of public health as a thematic in the training of many specialist clinical disciplines, even in the early educational stages of pre-registration programmes. Cuba, in parallel, promoted multispecialist contributions to its *Consultorios Populares*, which, while firmly family doctor based, sought even in the 1960s to incorporate elements of polyclinics effectively into the country's incipient Health For All policies and projects.

More recently in Brazil, a similar approach has been central to post-1990 policies for a Unified Health System (SUS), with the 1993 Base Operating Rule (BOR) enshrining principles of universality, equity and integration through an approach to decentralisation based on the reformed polyclinic. As we shall see in Chapter 5, the Brazilian model means trying to integrate private sector specialists, including those from family medicine, usually on a sessional or daily basis, into community clinics contracted to provide service-specific universal healthcare programmes. In Brazil, healthcare management is at the level of its 5500-plus municipalities and the country is characterised by a scale of social and economic inequalities matched only by South Africa. In such a context the SUS core principle of participation has to mean the inclusion of private professionals just as much as it does that of community groups representing, for example, indigenous people's or women's rights. The BOR nationally determined capitation rates in Brazil apply across the board: to the multispecialist polyclinic and to the generic healthcare practitioners of the community healthcare centre. Family medicine is a significant feature in both, supplied often from one small cubicle in the former, pervading the premises of the latter.

The reformed polyclinic in Brazil, as elsewhere, is often seen as a governmental response to growing middle-class expectations for individualised treatments, but within an overall framework of public health policy and funding.[13] This is, for example, evident in the hybrid health system of Greece. Here, particularly in the main cities of Athens and Thessalonica, family medicine is not so much the gatekeeper of, as the conduit to, specialist care. Since 2001 the independent national agency for 30 separate social insurance funds (IKA), operating as an independent association and registered charity, has been accrediting individual family doctors in their private premises with exclusive referral rights to the multispecialist IKA centres. In the capital itself these polyclinics may have up to 80 doctors, including further general medical practitioners. The IKA developments are explicitly based on the old Soviet *Semashko* system, but this time in the modern era, using polyclinics to guarantee nationally prescribed standards of care in the community, in this case for 5.5 million premium-paying Greek employees under the auspices of the Ministry for Social Affairs.[14]

The IKA 'Hub and Spoke' model has its counterparts elsewhere, scattered across the globe from the nine professions in the San Joaquín Family Health Centre of Santiago, Chile, piloted by the Ministry of Health with support from the main Catholic University (*see* p.73), to the curious semi-State, semi-private

SingHealth Clinic companies of Singapore and their counterparts in Taiwan. The main concentration of polyclinic developments remains, of course, in and around Russia, but in its reformation, its orientation as an organisational coalition of provider specialists, invariably including family medicine, is emphatically client based and consumerist. The reformed polyclinic places a commercial value on family medicine. It aligns this with modernising pressures for partnership with the private sector and, as the above illustrations indicate, in the twenty-first century it is an organisational form that, given the right culture and circumstances, can still effectively make progress on global principles of primary healthcare as well as national strategies for public health improvement. For family medicine the polyclinic is no dinosaur. Although often regarded as an intermediate or transitional primary care organisation, its future development does offer the prospect of higher specialist status, private reward and partnerships, all within a new ethos of public trust and wellbeing.

District health system

Alongside the extended general practice, the district health system (DHS) is the other principal starting point for understanding primary care developments internationally and the future role of family medicine. In large part this is because of the central sponsorship of the WHO. The WHO has a long history in more than 30 countries of using DHS sites for trialling new clinical roles and epidemiological research in primary care across Asia, parts of South America and, of course, much of Africa.[15] Indeed, the DHS was the operational framework for the introduction of barefoot doctors across China, as well as local healthcare technicians in parts of Latin America, 'triple-trained' nurses in southern Africa, and retrained internists and paediatricians in the republics of central Asia.[16,17]

As these indicate, substitution for family medicine is a defining feature of the DHS. In the parts of the world where the DHS prevails as a frontline service, and sometimes even as a secondary point of referral, the family doctor is too expensive to both train and maintain, and therefore a scarce commodity. As a result, the role of the DHS family doctor is strategic and supervisory. In terms of physical location this role may even be sited alongside specialist sources of clinical and planning expertise, in a university hospital, as in Pretoria, or at the level of the 100-plus bed district general hospital as in Kenya and Uganda. The role may not even be a native one, not just occupied by an overseas recruit – for example, a European general medical practitioner on a short-term secondment, sabbatical or elective – but also created by external sponsorship.

For the DHS is popular with donors. It is a rational and altruistic approach. It looks good on paper, not least because while it draws on Scandinavian-style academic 'impact assessments' from health economics and environmental studies, it also recognises the requirement of responding to local priorities.[18,19] Indeed, in negotiating these priorities the DHS approach allows for the identification of both new needs and new resources. A multitude of microfinance schemes have been spawned by the DHS. Local insurance, extended risk pooling for funeral charges, user fees and mutual benefit cooperatives are just the beginnings of a list which demonstrates the range of such schemes that are often supported by non-governmental organisations (NGOs). For the latter, whether as local or international charities, life assurance companies or churches, these schemes supply income in states where public expenditure on health is often limited largely to hospital settings and may well, in total, amount to well under half of that spent nationally on medical care.

Accordingly, family medicine in the DHS is part of a public health movement. The family doctor as District Medical Officer or equivalent oversees populations of up to a quarter of a million people. Nurse-led health centres operate within their remit for 20–30 000 population units and first aid outposts and stations sustained by subsistence level dispensers and volunteers located at the village or neighbourhood levels. In this management capacity, family doctors see relatively few patients in person themselves. But they can bring a focus on prevention and, if necessary, on palliative care as well, joined with a concern for social issues and social capital development, and a holistic philosophy which respects not just the integrity of the individual but also that of the clan, the tribe and the customs of the indigenous way of life.

DHS and SWAp go together under the terms of global modernisation. The Sector-Wide Approach (SWAp) is, and seems likely to continue to be, the prerequisite and precondition for donor support whether by governments or aid agencies.[20] It seeks to bring coherence to the new confusion of different accountabilities. Recipients of external assistance must be able to demonstrate effective frameworks for public administration with probity, partnerships with NGOs and participation. Good governance and democratic government are mandatory aims and the DHS paves the way for both. In Uganda, for example, each level of the DHS has a different level of healthcare provision; each matches a local level of community, with each tier of management being directly elected either by, for example, the county or village, or by representatives of the subordinate tiers. A representative family doctor, at the fifth level, may help to steer the primary care activity, interventions and profile of the whole system. The role of family medicine becomes that of sectoral direction and public leadership, intimately related to macropolicies for state revival and rehabilitation.[21]

Accordingly, for family medicine in a DHS, the orientation is bureaucratic with modern managerial values. Accountabilities are formal and prescribed with delineated lines of executive control and cross-agency links. The agenda of the DHS family doctor influences and is influenced by counterpart professionals managing parallel district functions which cover, for example, the environment, employment, production and economic development. Horizontal and, more particularly, vertical relationships can be drawn clearly and, if necessary to meet donor demands, diagrammatically. In systemic terms, family medicine becomes part of the throughput process. Where in other organisational models for primary care it would clearly be seen as an important input, in the DHS the doctor is key to the conversion of other inputs. These are localised combinations of funds, traditions, gifts, data, drugs, volunteers and, significantly, all informal intelligence and information, converted into outputs for increased immunisation and screening, reduced mortality and, above all, popular compliance with modern medical practices and procedures.

Family medicine fulfils this role admirably. Its professional status and clinical credibility qualify it for formal management, but more important, in the DHS its pastoral values and liberal principles position it ideally to harness alternative informal sources of healing, herbal remedies, historic treatments and therapies.

Moreover, because of these qualities, as the twenty-first century gathers pace so too do the ideas behind the DHS. No longer just the preserve of poorer countries, its potential for social capital and inclusion means that family medicine as a strategic force is increasingly recognised by such powerful policy analysts and advocates as the Health Systems Trust (in South Africa[22]), Nuffield Institute (UK) and several International Development Ministries in Western Europe. Ideologically at least it has a political and global future.

Community development agency

The other side of the coin to the DHS for family medicine, because it is grass-roots rather than government and governance based, is the community development agency. This is at least as political as the DHS in its motivation, and both are pivotal elements in local and national regeneration programmes. As a location for family doctors the community development agency is overwhelmingly at its strongest within the global region encompassed by the powerful and independently constituted Pan American Health Organization (PAHO). Throughout such countries as Colombia, Bolivia, Peru, Brazil, Argentina and even parts of Canada (e.g. Quebec, Ontario), the community health centre or clinic is emerging as an engine driving forward participatory democracy. Fostered by universal egalitarian movements and the slogans of citizenship and civil society, local ownership and management of primary care and its new organisations are regarded, in much of Latin America at least, as being at the heart of human rights and the restoration of national identities following periods of political unrest which have often meant military conflicts and even civil war.

In this context, such professional disciplines as family medicine are being both revived and redefined. The terminology is different. Under strong Cuban influence, GPs in, for example, Venezuela and Nicaragua practise what is now called 'integrated social medicine'. Social care and control is as significant here as clinical interventions, with doctors required to work and sometimes live alongside local women's groups, volunteers, auxiliaries, seniors' representatives and, not infrequently, outposted students and researchers from socially conscientious universities (e.g. Miguel del Lima in Peru, Simon Bolivar in Caracas) as well. Management ostensibly is by the people for the people. Indeed, often the origins of the community health committee in such places as Vietnam and Eritrea date back to nominated members of popular resistance movements or revolutions.[23,24]

Participation and empowerment are the watchwords. Family medicine signifies a popular entitlement, with regular household health needs assessments undertaken to ensure that, especially in poorer areas and among ethnic minorities, there is full and continuous access to its facilities. The PAHO approach is mirrored by developments elsewhere in the world for aboriginal peoples, with, for example, both New Zealand and Australia steadily transferring budgetary responsibilities to Maori and Torres Strait Islander community groups respectively for primary care provision and management over the past decade. Guinea, parts of Mexico and Indonesia, and southern Costa Rica, where the Chirripo tribes live, are further illustrations of the growth of family medicine in recent years within the context of new community development agencies.

For family medicine this context contains risks as well as opportunities. Peru is a beacon site in global terms for public participation, and its 2000-plus service outlets managed by community health committees (CLAS) have demonstrated real value for money in terms specific to patient satisfaction, prescribing and public health improvement.[25] Their standard seven-person steering group usually contains a family doctor as clinical director with three elected and three locally appointed lay representatives each charged with a communal responsibility for addressing an agreed local health priority. It sounds wonderful and sometimes it is, with women especially released into new roles and rights. But nationwide there remain considerable inequities; local management can be both inefficient and even corrupt, and national priorities and government can be undermined. With religious groups to the fore the community development agency can strengthen some social structures but may diminish others, with the result that family medicine is viewed as partisan or even marginal, associated only with the lower socioeconomic classes and alienated from other doctors and healthcare professions. Even in Finland, where the community development model for health and social care is firmly under municipal control, by 2003 over half of local authorities had failed to achieve accreditation for their primary care management mechanisms. Argentina, Slovakia and Colombia are other countries where we found that the decentralisation programmes have encountered similar difficulties.

In this model of primary care the orientation is communal. The organisational structure and process is that of a network. The community development agency is one of many with multiple relationships, often fluid and overlapping, held together by personal associations and ideological affiliations and operating for family medicine most effectively when a sense of common cause is evident. Such a cause will be expressed, as in Brazil, Peru and Venezuela, by large gatherings in the form of regional and national health assemblies or local citizens' forums. Sometimes, as with ForoSalud in Lima, these can all too readily be identified exclusively with (or even highjacked by) the political opposition and the threat of a coup and an alternative government. The advocacy role of the family doctor is subsumed within political activism and governments can feel compelled to respond authoritatively through restrictive laws and reduced funds. The emergent theoretical concepts of regulatory capture and resource dependency mean that in practice, for example in the Mexican provinces of Oaxaco[26] and Pachuca, the functions of family medicine are performed by poorly paid government workers each operating to standard ministerial procedures and programmes. Many of the local *Casas de Salud* have been taken into the national insurance agency and family medicine is reduced to a one-year live-in pre-qualifying experience for junior doctors undertaking a compulsory period of community service. Family medicine can easily become both champion and casualty in the community development agency.

Franchised outreach

This organisational type stands alone. It is primary healthcare in that family medicine is a frontline service, but it is not primary healthcare in its non-compliance with the principles of the classic WHO Alma Ata Declaration in 1978. Neither equity nor participation are formative factors in the franchising of services most often from and to hospitals, often as business developments in the marketplace. Competition and choice are the core economic values. Specialist family medicine here normally belongs to the private professional entrepreneur, and where in the preceding examples power has been devolved to communities or provider teams, in this case it is unequivocally and directly with the payers. Outreach family medicine under franchise is most evident across several countries of eastern Asia, and although it may be generous to regard it as an ideal type it is nevertheless an international phenomenon.

In Hong Kong, two-thirds of primary care is provided privately. The private sector also dominates the supply side in India. In Taiwan and Japan, the plethora of private and public insurance companies make their payments on the basis of consultation rates, based almost exclusively on hospital activity and expenditure. Thailand's contracting units for primary care also offer managed care franchise options to both private professional consortia and hospital corporations. China's cities are now dominated by fee-for-service facilities, and in their profile they look remarkably like many urban conurbations in such European countries as Germany and Greece. Recent research indicates many international parallel developments for family medicine in respect of this model.[27–32]

In all these locations family medicine is sourced from secondary care. It may well even be located in a clinic within a general hospital or, as in parts of Greece, the family doctor may receive private referral rights and fees from public hospitals. Regulation of family medicine as a private practice is often relatively minimal, with the title of general practitioner detached from vocational education programmes or requirements and claimed by many. When the contract from the insurer goes to a newly autonomous hospital organisation as a trust or foundation with public health management responsibilities then, as in Hong Kong and Singapore and prospectively even in England and Scotland, family medicine becomes another outpatient clinic sifting demand and providing preventive health promotion programmes.

Although, as in the case of The Philippines, there are exceptions, in ideal-type mode the franchised outreach is usually quasi-institutional in its values. It operates increasingly effectively in today's world as a modern virtual organisation. As such, its features are strong selective corporate objectives, centralised strategic direction and support services, semi-autonomous delivery units, internally regulated mechanisms and several different types of service outlet as business or cost centres. In reality, family medicine is both fragmented and fragile in this model, dependent on a combination of public prosperity and confidence, hospital consultants' goodwill and favour, and corporate or community sponsors. Not surprisingly, such a combination can often leave family medicine fending for itself. Turkey and The Philippines are two examples of countries where, for most people, family medicine is now no more than the small, individual private practice.

Organisational developments

Defining the different organisational developments taking place in relation to family medicine is important, because with a new century has come a new focus on the organisation rather than the person or the profession as the perceived unit of care. This perspective is essentially a political one. It recognises that virtually everywhere modern governments are looking to new organisational vehicles for the implementation of their policies as they seek to exercise national and local stewardship roles in public health. Organisational innovation offers the prospect of circumventing vested interests and professional or positional power in moving towards the goal which one WHO commentator has called the 'public choice' model of policy making in primary care.[33]

Describing the different organisational developments taking place in relation to family medicine as 'ideal types' is, of course, to acknowledge that none of the six models detailed above actually exists as described. This is not the purpose of 'ideal types'. In practice, they overlap, distort and merge. While individually distinct, all have some elements of each other. The most recent organisation to emerge, the managed care enterprise for example, emulates both the gatekeeping role of the extended general practice and the connections made in the district health system. There is, of course, no pure organisational form and no longer is there a pecking order between the different types. Each model belongs to its particular space in time and context.

Organisational typology

Nevertheless, as Table 2.1 demonstrates, from a global perspective, a genuine typology of actual primary care organisations can be postulated.

Table 2.1 Global typology of primary care organisational developments

Organisational type	Structure and process	Value base	Service focus	Location (examples)	Endpoint
Extended general practice	Simple, partnership	Normative	Registered patient list	Health centre	Patient
Managed care enterprise	Complex, stakeholder	Calculative	Target groups	Physicians group	User
Reformed polyclinic	Coalition, divisional	Commercial	Medical conditions	Multispecialist clinic	Client
District health system	Hierarchic, administrative	Executive	Public health improvement	General hospital	Populations
Community development agency	Association, network	Affiliative	Local populations	Health stations	Citizen
Franchised outreach	Quasi-institutional, virtual	Remunerative	Payers	Private, hospital premises	Customer

This summary (above) indicates the role of 'ideal type' descriptions in providing both a framework for comparative international analysis[34] and the basis for future scenario planning and theoretical definition in respect of family medicine. The six organisational developments are clearly different to the extent that, on some points, they seem diametrically opposed, with family medicine oscillating, for example, from the poor to the prosperous in terms of its patronage. But there are also several shared features or issues. Family medicine everywhere is being practised in larger organisations. These organisations are more flexible and less fixed over time. Generally, personal care is more at a premium and service recipients are increasingly of a collective identity. Monopolies are giving way to mixed economies of providers and payers, with family doctors (and others) deeply engaged in the emergence and creation of both. As disease profiles and drugs regimes change, family medicine everywhere is also more about maintenance and less about cure, with educative and executive roles increasing in response to requirements for more effective prevention, health promotion and rehabilitation. As a result, family medicine in all its forms is essential community care, with its particular denomination depending on local customs and conditions.

The different endpoint perspectives on family medicine and its future demonstrate the necessity of cultural fit. The extended general practice refers to 'patients'. The managed care enterprise has 'users' (or consumers) and the polyclinic receives 'clients'. The district health system is epidemiological in its population focus on named neighbourhoods, villages and townships, while it is the 'citizen' whose cause is advanced by the community development agency. This leaves the franchised primary care outreach organisation with, at best, its 'customers' or rather more likely such colloquial consumerist alternatives as 'punters' and 'price tags'.

It is clear that family medicine has many futures and more than one set of directions. Primary care itself is a political discourse. Its organisational developments reflect changes in power, policies, personalities and principles across societies where the status and significance of the family itself has become dynamic. Laws enshrine its sanctity in Bolivia and secularise its size in China: the generalist medical professional has to operate in very different worlds. Yet despite this spectrum of perspectives the relational issues may be seen to remain the same. The future role of the family doctor will be, as now and as before, to harness for the purposes of health all the positive relationships at the patient's disposal. In the chapters that follow we examine four international case exemplars of each of our six organisational models in order to understand in more detail the different ways in which these purposes may be achieved.

References

1 WONCA Europe (2002) *The European Definition of General Practice/Family Medicine.* Barcelona: WHO Europe Office.
2 Bivol G, Curocichin G, Sutnick A et al. (2002) Development of family medicine education in Moldova with Carelift International. *Education for Health.* 15(2): 202–14.
3 Koppel A, Meisar K, Valtonen H et al. (2003) Evaluation of primary health care reform in Estonia. *Social Science and Medicine.* 56: 2461–6.
4 Batterham R, Southern D, Appleby N et al. (2002) Construction of a GP integration model. *Social Science and Medicine.* 54: 1225–41.
5 Boelan C, Haq V, Hunt M et al. (2002) *Improving Health Systems: the contribution of family medicine.* Geneva: WONCA.

6 Cabiedes L, Guillen A (2002) Adopting and adapting managed competition: health care reform in southern Europe. *Social Science and Medicine*. **52**: 1205–17.

7 Flood C (2000) *International Health Care Reform. A legal, economic and political analysis.* London: Routledge.

8 Mills A, Brugha R, Hanson K et al. (2002) What can be done about the private health care sector in low income countries? *WHO Bulletin*. **80**(4): 325–30.

9 Reich M (2002) Reshaping the state from above, from within, from below: implications for public health. *Social Science and Medicine*. **54**: 1669–75.

10 Benson J (2001) The impact of privatisation on access in Tanzania. *Social Science and Medicine*. **52**: 1903–15.

11 Barrientos A, Lloyd-Sherlock P (2000) Reforming health insurance in Argentina and Chile. *Health Policy Plan*. **15**(4): 417–23.

12 Santana P (2002) Poverty, social exclusion and health in Portugal. *Social Science and Medicine*. **55**: 33–45.

13 Aravjo J, Barbosa J (2000) Decentralising the health sector: issues in Brazil. *Health Policy*. **52**: 113–27.

14 Tountas Y, Karnaki P, Pavi E (2002) Reforming the reform: the Greek national health system in transition. *Health Policy*. **62**: 15–29.

15 Tollman S, Zwi A (2000) Health systems reform and the role of field sites based upon demographic and health surveillance. *WHO Bulletin*. **78**: 125–34.

16 Woodward D, Drager N, Beaglehole R et al. (2001) Globalisation and health: a framework for analysis and action. *WHO Bulletin*. **79**: 875–81

17 Widdus R (2001) Public-private partnerships for health: their main targets, their diversity, and their future directions. *WHO Bulletin*. **79**: 713–20.

18 Niessen L, Grijseels E, Rutten F (2000) The evidence-based approach in health policy and health care delivery. *Social Science and Medicine*. **51**: 859–69.

19 Johns D (2001) Health and development in South Africa: from principles to practice. *Development*. **44**(1): 122–8.

20 Hill P (2002) The rhetoric of sector-wide approaches for health development. *Social Science and Medicine*. **55**: 1725–37.

21 Jeppsson A (2002) SWAp dynamics in a decentralised context: experiences from Uganda. *Social Science and Medicine*. **55**: 2053–60.

22 Saunders D, Chopra M (2001) Implementing comprehensive and decentralised health systems. *International Journal of Integrated Care*. **1**(2): 1–13.

23 Jowett M, Contoyannis P, Vinh N (2003) The impact of public voluntary health insurance on private health care expenditures in Vietnam. *Social Science and Medicine*. **56**: 333–42.

24 Kloos H (1998) Primary health care in Ethiopia under three political systems: community participation in a war-torn society. *Social Science and Medicine*. **46**: 505–22.

25 Iwami M, Petchey R (2002) A CLAS act? Community-based organisations, health service decentralisation and primary care development in Peru. *Journal of Public Health Medicine*. **44**(4): 246–51.

26 Zakus J (1998) Resource dependency and community participation in primary health care. *Social Science and Medicine*. **47**: 927–39.

27 Gould D (1998) A survey of the Hong Kong health sector: past, present and future. *Social Science and Medicine*. **47**: 927–39.

28 Lui T, Chin S (2002) An analysis of insurance purchasing decisions with national health insurance in Taiwan. *Social Science and Medicine*. **55**: 755–74.

29 Ikegami N, Creighton Campbell J (1999) Health care reform in Japan: the virtues of muddling through. *Health Affairs*. **18**(3): 56–75.

30 Wibulpolprasert S, Pongpaiboon P (2001) Economic dynamics and health: lessons from Thailand. *Development*. **44**(1): 99–107.

31 Riemer-Hommel P (2002) The changing nature of contracts in German health care.

Social Science and Medicine. **55**: 1447–55.

32 Liaropoulos L, Tragakes E (1998) Public/private financing in the Greek health care system: implications for equity. *Health Policy.* **43**(2): 153–69.

33 Scruton R (2000) *WHO, What and Why? Transnational government, legitimacy and the World Health Organization.* London: Institute of Economic Affairs.

34 Light D (1997) Community health care: the limits of countervailing powers to meet the health care needs of the twenty-first century. *Journal of Health Politics, Policy and Law.* **22**(1): 106–45.

Chapter 3

The extended general practice

Introduction

The extension of general practice is more about the growing reach of a philosophy of care than it is about any increase in the size of buildings or even personnel. The philosophy is rooted in relationships and their potential to contribute to health and healthcare. Accordingly, in contemporary policy developments within the NHS in the UK, it has been a number of primary care organisations that have championed the cause of relational healthcare as a counterweight to the thrust of the evidence-based medicine (EBM) proponents who have propelled forward the managed care enterprise, especially in North America. The argument tends to polarise over which of the two burgeoning ideologies comes first, with the extended general practice offering an operational framework founded on relational perspective.[1]

This has attracted like-minded and motivated primary care practitioners to the side of family doctors in unprecedented numbers. As the size of the general practice team and premises has extended so too has the service focus, from individual patients to special needs target groups and then to the aggregate registered lists of a practice as a single and coherent local population. The challenge is that of applying past principles of longitudinal, comprehensive and personal care to the interventions required by this new scale of responsibilities. This challenge is the greater because of the opposition it encounters, not just from exclusive EBM advocates, but also from those, like some statutory health and local authorities, who feel that their traditional territories are being invaded. Many clinical specialisms, conditions, and nursing and therapeutic roles – not to mention the monies that went with them – which were once the preserve of secondary care institutions and their medical consultants, are now firmly in the domain of the extended general practice.

The following case exemplars from Kangasala and Wimborne illustrate this transfer of functions especially well. The extended general practice is at heart interprofessional. But while it is no longer unidisciplinary, the family doctor or the general medical practitioner remains its pivotal person. The case exemplars from Anogia and Viseu highlight the continuing clinical development of the GP as provider. Alongside this development as a modern primary care organisation, it is this primary care professional who also leads the creation of the educational and executive capacity required in the assumption of public health and social and secondary care commissioning duties. Despite its origins as a small business directed by sometimes maverick independent entrepreneurs, it is hard to imagine, given all its strengths and levels of public trust, that the extended general practice will not be able to adapt to the legitimate governance demands of modern participatory democracies and flourish into the future, right across the planet.

Kangasala

'Even health economists never say a bad word about each other.' So we were advised, ever so slightly tongue in cheek, by a distinguished professor of health policy in Helsinki. He had generously agreed to brief us on the 2002–2008 countrywide modernising health project in Finland. 'We are a family more than a nation,' commented the Kangasala Health Centre Medical Director a few days later. The language of the Finnish reform process with its 'care chains' and 'service circles' is one that reflects a deep cultural conditioning in consensual decision making and developments. Inevitably the last have long but lasting lead-in times.

Management is a brokerage function between professions, politicians and the public. 'Blowing on the coals', another Finnish health policy professor called it at one of our workshop sessions. The role of central government, according to a civil servant responsible for the new primary care policies, is that of 'guidance by information', and civil servants are themselves termed 'counsellors'. In their brokerage role, the currency is not so much money as ideas, with proposals for decentralisation representing an amalgam of five different political parties' proposals. Each party is a constituent in the national government, each has elected municipal strongholds and each is 'affiliated' to one of Finland's major university medical schools. In many ways Finland felt the most sophisticated of all the States we studied. Within Europe it has been the country recognised as the frontrunner in cross-sectoral social and economic policies deliberately designed for health improvement.[2]

Certainly its political environment and social context permitted the largest general practices we encountered between 2002 and 2005. The target norm nationally is a health centre with 20 general medical practitioners, each with a registered list of 1500–1600 local patients. This is four times the size of the English counterpart, where partnership 'splits' and consequent organisational turnover remain an everyday *angst*. In the UK, placing 20 frontline doctors together would be a cultural anathema with almost certainly disastrous consequences. In Finland, these new groupings into municipally based primary care organisations represent essential 'modernisation'. They are explicitly seen as the vehicles for maintaining popular 'trust' and 'respect', not only in the local health system but in Finland itself and all it stands for.

The Kangasala Health Centre in the centre of the country actually has 28 general medical practitioners, with 82 rather than the usual 60 beds.* Its catchment population similarly is a little over the standard 30 000 figure which is

---

* The present tense is used through the exemplar case study accounts in this and the next five chapters. This is simply for ease of narrative. Readers will realise that, especially at local levels, services are changing all the time and the data provided in my narrative attempts to be accurate, but only for the time at which it was collected, during the 2002–05 period. Within this context the author accepts full responsibility for all errors and omissions.

being used to rationalise or reduce the number of health centres in Finland's 481 municipalities to about half that total. Under the auspices of 'decentralisation', the post-2002 Finnish reforms are resulting in mergers, especially in the more remote northern and eastern parts of the country, and the advent for the first time of multi-municipality regional councils. The Finnish decentralisation is not so much about localism and geographic sovereignty as it is concerned with the integration of communities and their legitimate representatives. Some of these in terms of, for example the private sector and higher education institutes, are relatively new to the national health system.

At Kangasala all these elements are in evidence. Nominated as an exemplar of the extended general practice by both the municipally funded National Research and Development Institute (STAKES) and the Ministry of Health in Helsinki, the Kangasala Health Centre has a management board comprising seven elected members from five municipal authorities (including three from the centre's host area), plus a lead nurse and dentist, with the GP clinical director and general manager sharing chief executive responsibilities. Within the centre the overall operational control of service provision is exercised by the general medical practitioners on the basis of their levels of both education and specialist skills. The former is based on a minimum 12-year period for general medicine, with three of the first six pre-registration years, for both doctors and nurses, being based in non-hospital community settings. In relation to the senior status afforded to the doctors at Kangasala, their specialisms include, *inter alia*, minor casualty, orthopaedics, gastroscopy, paediatrics, psychiatry, obstetrics, rehabilitation, palliative care and, for the entire local population of catchment municipalities, occupational health.

These extensions to general practice attract additional 'buy-ins' both from other professions and from the public. As a result the primary healthcare team stretches well beyond the physical premises through, for example, attached Red Cross ambulances, research and educational programmes with the local University of Tampere, and shared care protocols with the new (German) privately financed and trade union-supported Coxa Ltd diagnostic and treatment centre. At Kangasala the other professionals include four psychologists, eight physiotherapists and eight laboratory technicians, 16 dentists and dental assistants, two mental health and a small group of generic social workers, plus a whole range of public health, community and acute care nurses. Although, by law, the individual can choose and access directly clinical specialists, in practice the extended general practice is in a gatekeeper role for both secondary and social care. Both are combined at the commissioning level of elected municipal management. It is the municipality too that owns and majority funds (about 70%) the health centre. These funds are augmented at Kangasala with a 20% contribution to local service developments from patients themselves through, for example, registration, weekend and night-time call-out fees, plus payments from those who opt to contribute 1% of their income through a designated charity tax, and employers' occupational health contracts.

Services are both comprehensive and to a high standard. The 1972 Primary Health Care Act in Finland was a global forerunner in terms of locating community health and development responsibilities with primary care. Kangasala Health Centre itself hosts no fewer than 36 public health nurses and six environmental health and animal welfare officers, while in terms of inpatient care, GPs lead teams

dedicated to rapid recovery and maximum bed utilisation through intensive rehabilitation and domiciliary support programmes (e.g. for hip replacement patients).
Accordingly, while a length of stay may be six months, two to three nights is the
norm; and such preventive measures as biannual mammograms after the age of
50, five-yearly health checks for women and regular mandatory examinations for
men from 19 years onwards, mean many admissions are planned and proactive.
Remarkably, when we visited the extended general practice at Kangasala, it had a
total of 293 full- and part-time staff; and the doctors themselves are, of course,
salaried and public service employees.

Finland[†]	
1 Capital city:	Helsinki
2 Demographic factors:	
Population size (million)[a]	5.25 (2005)
Age profile[a]	5.3% (aged < 5), 15.9% (aged 65 and over) (2005)
Ethnicity[b]	Finn 93.4%; Swede 5.7%; Russian 0.4%; Estonian 0.2%
3 Socioeconomic factors:	
GDP per capita (International $)[c]	26 614 (2002)
Health expenditure per capita (International $)[c]	1943 (2002)
Health expenditure per GDP[c]	7.3% (2002)
Main industry[b]	Metal products; electronics; machinery and scientific instruments; shipbuilding; pulp and paper; foodstuffs; chemicals; textiles; clothing
4 Health factors:	
Life expectancy at birth[c]	79.0 (M 75.0/F 82.0) (2003)
Five main causes of death (rate per 100 000 population)[d]	Diseases of circulatory system, 406.36; neoplasms*, 202.32; external causes, 131.23; diseases of respiratory system, 74.32; mental disorders, 62.42 (2002, ICD 10 used, coverage rate 100%)
5 Organisational factors:	
Primary care model	Municipality-based health centres with extended multiprofessional general practice teams

Resources (health personnel)[e]	31.9 physicians/10 000 pop. (2003); 221.9 nurses and midwives/10 000 pop. (2003)
Financing[f]	Local taxation; out-of-pocket payments; State subsidies; National Health Insurance (NHI) funds; few voluntary health insurance schemes
Lead primary care practitioners	GPs

Policy priorities

A *Responsive combinations of health and social care*
  Local needs-led approach; shifting mental health to primary care
B *Partnerships, collaboration and participation*
  Promotion of the combination of health and social care through the merger and collaboration of municipalities and health centres
C *Management*
  Single unified records for health and social care for greater equity, efficiency and integration of primary and secondary care
D *Human resources*
  Integrated educational programmes for multipurpose practice nurses
E *Research*
  Primary care research centres at universities

* Neoplasms include both cancers and benign growths.
† The country profiles are designed to give readers a snapshot of the national context for each exemplar of primary care. The public health statistics are largely based on the latest WHO publications with some exceptions where this is outdated and alternative and valid domestic figures are available. The lists of sources are set out at the end of each chapter.

Viseu

Only once beyond the shores of the UK in our worldwide search for model primary care organisations, did we witness facilities that might be regarded as even remotely a match for those at Kangasala. These were once again in an extended general practice and once again in the centre of the country: Portugal. Located inland and midway between the ancient capital of Coimbra and the modern Atlantic Ocean city of Oporto, Viseu Health Centre is a superb site for a modern primary care development. Purpose built and in pristine condition, in physical terms it is the classic expression of the strategies for primary healthcare that, particularly during the 1997–2000 period, grew out of the Portuguese Interior Ministry's modernising post-1995 policies for public protection.[3]

At the heart of these was the idea of integration, underpinned by the economic necessity of more efficient resource utilisation. This integration is, accordingly, both managerial and professional. For the former it means the overall performance management of local health systems (LHS) by central government with, under the terms of Law 60 in 2003, a deregulated diversity of mixed-status provision subject to overall monitoring by five administrative regions, and operational support in terms of legal, financial and human resources management, at subregional or district level. Within the LHS are not only private and voluntary agencies but the public services for education, training, employment and welfare. The aim is that at a health centre such as that of Viseu you should be able to access directly, if necessary, pathways to your social security payment, your job skills course or your child care benefits. And *vice versa* in terms of pathways to primary healthcare if you go, for example, into the local job or adult learning centre.

Integration in professional terms means a major focus on teamwork and positive discrimination towards private practice alongside public service. Teamwork figures prominently in the initial and final stages of medical, nursing and social work qualifying curricula, which are of six years' duration for doctors and four years for the other two caring professions. The 2003 legislation encouraged the franchising or contracting out of primary healthcare services to private agencies following the perceived success of the Alpha Project in Lisbon and the appointment of a health minister with strong links to European private hospital companies (e.g. Group Mello).

At the Viseu Health Centre the twin approach to managerial and professional integration is clearly evident. Centre coordination is provided by a triumvirate: GP clinical director, administrator and lead nurse. All service programmes have a dual GP/nurse leadership with most being delivered on set days of the week: maternity on Monday, diabetes on Tuesday, etc. With statutory social care responsibilities incorporated into the role of the health centre at Viseu, the contribution of a qualified social assistant is written into each programme. Other professional services, usually on a sessional basis, include those of the nutritionist, oral hygienist and physiotherapist. For a 32 000 population – 4000 above the new national norm – Viseu has an establishment of 16 general medical practitioners, six of whom work mostly from local branch surgeries supported by the health centre. It also supports closely the local *Misericórdias*, the traditional and Catholic faith-based charities which offer the equivalent of long-term nursing home and short-term rehabilitative care. The Viseu Health Centre is at the forefront of the drive by the GP-led national Institute of Health Quality (IQS) to lift standards in primary care through accreditation of post-qualifying courses for doctors in general medicine and the publication of local audits. It uses a capitation-based payments system based on weighted reimbursements for those under two and over 65 to encourage registered lists. This is viewed as an essential part of the modernisation of a national health system previously based on public hospital catchment areas of minimum 60 000 population and relatively unregulated individual practitioner premises.

The extended general practice in Portugal still has a long way to go. It is beset by resource shortfalls, a lack of effective general management and cultural conservatism. When we visited Viseu, for example, 8000 of the local 32 000 population remained unregistered with a GP. Only five of the doctors had made a full-time employment commitment to the centre, which had yet to attract sessions from, for example, local dermatologists, ear, nose and throat specialists, psychologists and dentists. They remained fully committed to their own separate businesses. Whereas Finland lays claim to the largest proportion of community nurses in Europe, Portugal still has one of the smallest, and even at

Viseu the reluctance of social workers to practise in a medical setting meant there was only one social assistant, while nationally the ratio remains at 1:50 000. Similarly, for Portugal as a whole, such modernising policies as shared formularies with community pharmacies and registered GP lists with capitation payments apply to less than 10% of the people; and 30% still prefer to access their healthcare direct from hospital emergency rooms even in poorer urban areas.

Nevertheless, the Viseu Health Centre is an emergent example of the extended general practice and its potential. As at Kangasala, it is a gatekeeper to both secondary and social care, with counselling services among its portfolio of public health promotion, preventive and treatment programmes, with modern technology, quality and communications prominent in its development. Unlike at Kangasala, however, this development at Viseu is not taking place within a unified and ordered municipal framework, but rather less predictably, as part of a mixed economy of provider initiatives that encompass national projects and private professional enterprise. It is both haphazard and dynamic and, as such, it seems to suit the extended general practice model with its inherent and individualistic capacity to respond flexibly to both opportunity and societal demands.

Portugal	
1 Capital city:	Lisbon
2 Demographic factors:	
Population size (million)[a]	10.50 (2005)
Age profile[a]	5.3% (aged < 5), 17.1% (aged 65 and over) (2005)
Ethnicity[b]	Homogeneous Mediterranean stock; citizens of black African descent less than 100 000; since 1990 some East Europeans
3 Socioeconomic factors:	
GDP per capita (International $)[c]	18 376 (2002)
Health expenditure per capita (International $)[c]	1702 (2002)
Health expenditure per GDP[c]	9.3% (2002)
Main industry[b]	Textiles and footwear; wood pulp, paper and cork; metals; oil refining; chemicals; fish canning; rubber and plastic products; ceramics; electronics and communications equipment; transportation equipment; ship construction and refurbishment; wine; tourism

4 Health factors:
   Life expectancy at birth[c]   77.0 (M 74.0/F 81.0) (2003)
   Five main causes of death
   (rate per 100 000 population)[d]   Diseases of circulatory system,
                                             395.44; neoplasms, 219.78; external
                                           causes, 94.33; diseases of respiratory
                                           system, 89.21; endocrine,
                                           nutritional and metabolic diseases,
                                           48.07 (2002, ICD 10 used, coverage
                                           rate 100%)

5 Organisational factors:
   Primary care model   Relatively large health GP-based centres for about 30 000 population with inpatient beds and 24-hour care
   Resources (health personnel)[e]   32.6 physicians/10 000 pop. (2002); 40.3 nurses and midwives/10 000 pop. (2003)
   Financing[g]   General taxation for regional public services plus employee and employer contributions for social health insurance and out-of-pocket payments; voluntary private health insurance funds; mutual funds; external funds (e.g. EU)
   Lead primary care practitioners   GPs (with nurse pairings)

Policy priorities
A *Partnerships and participation*
   Development of new forms of collaboration between public and private, and health and social sectors, including involvement of charitable NGO '*Misericórdias*' and commercial companies
B *Management and regulation*
   Establishment of benchmarking and quality assurance for primary care, national standard information systems and clinical governance procedures
C *Integrated public services*
   Common access to health, welfare, education and employment rights and services through overarching domestic strategies, multiprofessional developments and shared information

Anogia

Crete is not Greece and Greece is not what it was. Once the most sophisticated of ancient civilisations, its public services now are so varied and variable, so informally (and sometimes even corruptly) organised and so different in practice to their formal expressions in policy[4] that it is impossible to say that there is a coherent national model of primary care. Across its multiple islands and mainland exist every form of healthcare finance yet devised: local and national taxation, private fees and payments in kind, occupational and social insurance, donor funding and European Union grants; and so it goes on. One of our interviewees, a big city health region president told us, not surprisingly and rather ironically, that 'accountability is still rather a new idea in Greece', where, in his view it still scores 'zero'. Another eminent professor explained that laws in Greece are essentially 'permissive not prescriptive'. After all, of the 210 public primary healthcare centres proposed for urban areas when the Greek National Health Service (ESY) legislation was first passed in 1983, none has actually been built.[5] To return to the wisdom of our city president: for him the Greek health environment comprises continuously overlapping 'circles of influence', usually with medical academics and financial entrepreneurs at the centre, with overall direction coming from those that are successful in 'pulling strings from behind the curtains'.

The principal policy adviser on primary care at the Ministry of Health put it more bluntly: 'We have lots of laws but are without the mechanisms for enforcing rules.' One chief architect of the post-2001 Greek modernisation, which is based on a plan for the merger of existing service outlets into 4000 GP-led and multiprofessional health centres countrywide within 17 regional health systems *(Periferiaka Systimata Ygias)*, blamed excessive 'fragmentation' and factionism for their patchy implementation. He echoed the city President's view that 'in Greece we belong to different countries'.

One of these 'countries' is clearly Crete, and what all our interviewees recognised was that on this Mediterranean island, and perhaps only here, the Greek vision for modern primary care genuinely prevails. That it does so in a country where everybody is 'my very good friend' is, of course, largely down to personal influence and local politics. The extended general practices of Crete have their roots in the relationships of a local doctor brought up as a child with GPs in Scandinavia. As an adult he moved into academic research collaborations with GPs in northern Europe and management education projects with health executives in the UK. All these influences come together in the creation of the Anogia Health Centre up in the mountains in the middle of Crete, 38 kilometres from the capital Heraklion. All our sources agreed it is the 'best' extended general practice in the country.

Because of its largely rural setting it serves only 9000 people, all on a single registered list with the health centre itself. The total is well below national norms because of the terrain and dispersed population. There are eight GPs in two tiers. Four are of 'specialist' status having completed a four-year post-qualifying programme in addition to the initial six-year pre-registration period. Anogia Health Centre is regionally funded and administered, but via the principal regional hospital in Heraklion. This arrangement is reflected in the clinical profile and focus of the specialist GP training. It includes, for example, ward-based periods of three to six months in intensive care, orthopaedics, cardiology, ophthalmology and internal medicine. There are proposals to extend the programme to six years, reflecting the health centre's growing role in the provision, via its specialist GPs, of radiology, emergency medicine and even chemotherapy services. The centre has five short-term inpatient beds and is open 24 hours a day all year round.

The Anogia Health Centre is doctor-dependent. There are only three qualified nurses on the staff, as well as one paediatrician and a laboratory technician. A chapel stands at the entrance. The centre has no volunteers, but it regularly receives gifts and legacies. From our observations it would appear that the doctors do not usually have to pay for their drinks in Anogia. This cultural informality operates alongside a distinctive formality of stratified professional status designed to ensure scope for real career prospects and progression even within an extended general practice the size of Anogia. There are four grades of GP each reflecting higher clinical competence, qualifications, experience and complexity of morbidities that can be addressed by a responsible doctor. The centre director, a GP with 13 years' post-qualifying experience, is at another level on his own and his managerial responsibilities include the research leadership of the centre, which is formally a designated epidemiological unit of the University of Crete.

At the Anogia Health Centre, accordingly, the unique Greek respect and appreciation of the academic, the clinical and the cultural come together in its modern form of extended general practice. This means that a doctor in Anogia can hold the title of assistant professor, have a large consulting room with x-ray and imaging equipment, and happily use local herbal remedies as well to 'see off the evil eye within you and others'. (These are the actual words of one of the health centre doctors interviewed by our research team.)

Nationwide, around 44% of healthcare expenditure is in kind or out of pocket. At Anogia there are no figures, but it is probably higher, reflecting the strong traditional community ties and contributions. These seem to have pre-empted the scale of formal social work developments evident elsewhere in Europe. On Crete the four-person homecare teams each comprise a social worker, a community nurse and two domiciliary assistants. Every team is peripatetic and local authority managed. Each covers a 5000 population. Two teams use the Anogia Health Centre as a partner and a base. Both receive the majority of their funding via Brussels as a European Union initiative. It seems paradoxical in the country that has often enjoyed the longest life expectancies in Europe, at a time when public health movements are so insistently adopting social welfare, that the latter should require external sponsorship in Crete. Greece is a law unto itself, impossible to emulate, but at Anogia there is nevertheless a model of extended general practice in a rural area for the rest of us to learn from and admire.

Greece

1 Capital city:	Athens
2 Demographic factors:	
Population size (million)[a]	11.12 (2005)
Age profile[a]	4.6% (aged < 5), 18.2% (aged 65 and over) (2005)
Ethnicity[b]	Greek 98%; others 2%

3 Socioeconomic factors:
GDP per capita (International $)[c] 19 041 (2002)
Health expenditure per capita
(International $)[c]   1814 (2002)
Health expenditure per GDP[c]   9.5% (2002)
Main industry[b]   Tourism; food and tobacco
                                       processing; textiles; chemicals; metal
                                       products; mining

4 Health factors:
Life expectancy at birth[c]   79.0 (M 76.0/F 81.0) (2003)
Five main causes of death
(rate per 100 000 population)[d]   Diseases of circulatory system,
                                       470.56; neoplasms, 222.96; external
                                       causes, 76.28; diseases of respiratory
                                       system, 64.14; diseases of digestive
                                       system, 22.07 (2001, ICD 9 BTL
                                       used, coverage rate 90.2%)

5 Organisational factors:
Primary care model   GP-based medical centres, private
                                       practices and polyclinics
Resources (health personnel)[e]   45.3 physicians/10 000 pop. (2001);
                                       31.0 nurses and midwives/10 000
                                       pop. (1995)
Financing[h,i]   44% out-of-pocket payments
                                       (official, unofficial); general
                                       taxation; employer and employee
                                       contributions and government
                                       subsidies for social insurance
                                       schemes; voluntary private health
                                       insurance funds; European Union
Lead primary care practitioners   GPs

Policy priorities
A *Coverage*
  Expand primary care service forms of provision to increase utilisation
  and secure funding within NHS
B *Decentralisation*
  Transferring responsibility for primary care and monitoring role to 17
  regions
C *Partnerships and integration/networks*
  Promoting multiple payers and providers across sectors; partnerships
  with universities on management of health systems; and establishing
  primary care networks with single information and database systems

D *Management and governance*
  Establishing government stewardship role in public health with standard information system and new payment schemes
E *Human resources*
  Promoting internist retraining programmes

Wimborne

For the past decade, if measured by performance on the London government's performance indicators and targets, Dorset has been the leading health authority in England. The first to espouse the policies of a 'Primary Care-led National Health Service (NHS)'[6,7] in the early and mid-1990s, it has built its success on the foundations of extended general practices which, through the local coordination of service teams and employment contracts, effectively bring together the different family health services which comprise community pharmacy and nursing, general dental and optical services, and, of course, general medical practice.

The Quarterjack Surgery at Wimborne has epitomised the distinctive Dorset style over the past ten years. Readily accessible, modern and in a prominent market town centre position with excellent adjacent facilities, including public parking, it has a registered list of 13 500 patients. Named after one of the towers in the local minster it dates back to 1907. Its sense of local history and local service responsibility is palpable. It is also unequivocally a local business and a proactive one at that. Twenty-four-hour cover is provided for the local community hospital but charged on the basis of a commercial cooperative. Foreign tourists are welcomed but pay as fee-for-service private patients. A major pharmacy occupies part of the entrance area on a revenue-generating rental basis. There are private chargeable chiropody and physiotherapy services available. Finally, all of the GPs supply specialist services that attract local secondary care referral rates through the commissioning activities of the nearest NHS primary care trust.

Profit and income levels help drive the Quarterjack Surgery forward in its focus on teamwork, personal patient lists and pastoral care. In the English general practice, unlike elsewhere, the tensions between independent employment status and public service values seem to create a dynamic for continuous growth with the self-interest of general medical practice a constant challenge to exploit for NHS politicians and managers. Their encounters are never easy. I have been visiting the Quarterjack Surgery for over a decade and the negative refrain from different GP partners has never changed during this time: not enough resources, too much management; and not good enough management, a government that does not understand and, of course, excessive bureaucracy and insufficient freedom. The list never changes.

In the interview for this case study, one senior doctor echoed his predecessors down the years by asserting, once more, that if all the above were sorted out the extended general practice could reduce secondary care activity by 'at least 40%'. The purpose remains, for all the concerns and complaints, to extend the business by placing all 'low-risk and high-volume work in primary care'. The business is, of course, still a GP monopoly. There are eight doctors with local partnership status who are the proprietors of the Quarterjack Surgery. They are supported and protected by no fewer than eight receptionists, three more than the number of practice nurses. Three further GPs are paid as retainers with particular specialist skills and roles, including the support of special needs adults and children in a range of local educational and residential establishments. The whole service configuration is wrapped up in a single personal medical services contract, which the local primary care trust negotiates and monitors on behalf of the NHS and in accordance with its national priorities and performance indicators. Last year the Quarterjack Surgery achieved 1490 out of 1500 on the NHS 'balanced scorecard' of its Quality and Financial Framework,* placing it in the highest echelon of UK primary care. With this accolade, of course, came the highest level of remuneration. Wimborne headed the extended general practice overachievers which, some commentators believe, led to the government hastily bringing forward its review of the new terms for general medical services.[8,9]

At the Quarterjack this promise of a rethink was still not enough. The doctors do not like relying on sessional psychologists subcontracted from another NHS trust; or having to wait up to 11 weeks for their patients' hospital treatments; or depending on social workers from a local municipal authority to lead on child protection and domiciliary care cases. The in-house counsellor is no substitute and the health visitors remain separately supervised. During our research period there were proposals for a larger primary care organisation covering 24 000 people with two smaller general practices joining the Quarterjack. The stumbling block remained the requirement for 100% GP control – of a budget spiralling into several million pounds sterling with just a friendly fundraising League of Friends for community governance.

To the patient at the Quarterjack little of the local politics is apparent or matters. The waiting room is warm, comfortable and welcoming. So too are the well-equipped, computerised, clean and confidential personal consulting rooms. There are two staffed receptions as well as a self check-in system. This is being extended in 2005/06 to include hospital outpatient and inpatient appointments with a selection of up to five alternative provider locations on offer. The 'Caring for You' clinics number 17 in the weekly schedule and are comprehensive in their range, from preventive 'Smokestop' and 'Child Health Surveillance' to rehabilitative cardiac, diabetes and bereavement groups. The GPs list and publicise the same number of specialisms: from gastroenterology to school medicine. Internal referrals for sports injuries, minor surgery, osteopathic medicine, dermatology and women's health are so heavy that their 'lead' doctors now set aside one or more days in the week solely for their practice. The dedicated specialisms of the primary care nurses correspond directly to these clinical areas and they work to the responsible individual doctors on these days.

The 18-page Quarterjack brochure and its website are packed full of valuable information about its services, local facilities, and health and healthcare in general, with lots of good simple advice for self-help purposes. Twenty-five neighbourhoods are specifically mapped out as the Quarterjack territory and

---

* Quality and Outcomes Framework. See www.bma.org.uk

the 2004 brochure ends with an advert for a recommended funeral director. As an extended general practice it seems to do just about everything, at least within the physical constraints of its 1992 surgery premises.

So, to hear an interviewee describe the role of the modern British GP as 'a bit-part player' comes as something of a shock. The practice manager describes relationships with NHS managers at 'an all-time low' and under strain with other local community professionals. The term 'primary care' is treated with disdain: 'too malleable to be meaningful' and evidently seen as 'imprisoning' in its impact, paving the way for overwhelming NHS performance management and allegedly preventing the extended general practice reaching its potential.

And what is this assumed potential? Control of all the healthcare and public health resource of course. The extended general practice in this part of England strives ceaselessly for more power and people. It seems it will not be satisfied until the day when this includes the acute hospitals, the social workers and the pharmacists. To appease these demands and perhaps as a tease as well, policy makers in London are introducing a new organisational model for primary and secondary care relationships across England by the end of 2006. Entitled 'Practice-based Commissioning' its stated purpose is to extend both local choice and professional control of commissioning, bringing 'tangible benefits for patients' and 'high levels of clinical engagement'.[10] Predictably, at the Quarterjack it has already been dismissed as 'a step backwards, supplying the illusion of devolution while retaining central executive command'. The extended general practice is being left 'with all the micro-decision making' only. Whether true or not they do it very well.

England

1 Capital city:	London
2 Demographic factors:	
Population size (million)[a]	50.09 (2004)
Age profile[a]	5.7% (aged < 5), 16.0% (aged 65 and over) (2004)
Ethnicity[b]	White 91.3% (British 87.5%, Irish 1.2%, other white 2.6%); mixed 1.3%; Asian or Asian British 4.4% (Indian 2.0%, Pakistani 1.4%, Bangladeshi 0.5%, other Asian 0.5%); black or black British 2.2%
3 Socioeconomic factors:	
GDP per capita (International $)[c]	27 959 (UK, 2002)
Health expenditure per capita (International $)[c]	2160 (UK, 2002)
Health expenditure per GDP[c]	7.7% (UK, 2002)
Main industry[d]	Property and business services; retail; public administration and

		other services; construction; hotels and catering; education (2004)
4	Health factors:	
	Life expectancy at birth[e]	78.5 (M 76.2/F 80.7) (2002)
	Five main causes of death (rate per 100 000 population)[f]	Diseases of circulatory system, 389.27; neoplasms, 263.97; diseases of respiratory system, 142.32; diseases of digestive system, 47.26; external causes of morbidity and mortality, 31.62 (England and Wales total pop. 52 793 700 in 2003, ICD 10 used, coverage rate 100%)
5	Organisational factors:	
	Primary care model	General practices accountable to NHS primary care trusts
	Resources (health personnel)[a,g]	23.5 physicians/10 000 pop. (2004); 74.9 nurses and midwives/10 000 pop. (2004)
	Financing	National general taxation (majority); out-of-pocket payments (prescriptions and dental charges only for NHS); 10–12% private health insurance funds
	Lead primary care practitioners	GPs

Policy priorities[h,i]

A *Health improvement and protection*

  With special attention to the needs of the poorest people, those with long-term conditions and inequalities

B *Access*

  Faster access and reducing waiting through a wider range of first contact services, choice of providers, booking systems and better emergency care

C *Quality of care*

  Improved patient experience through effective standards and regulation

D *Capacity building and partnerships*

  Modernised systems in health and social care through IT investment, new staff contracts, best value including not-for-profit and private providers

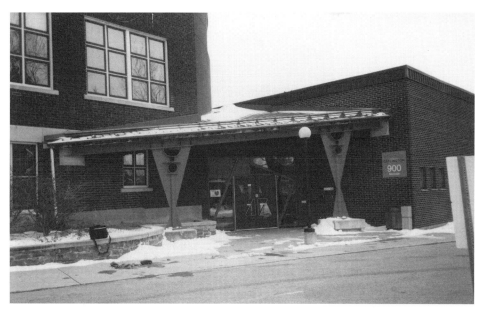

Figure 1 Kangasala, Finland.

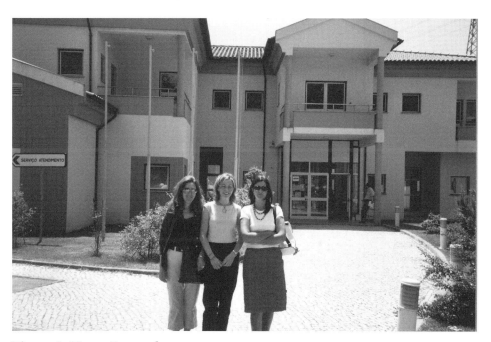

Figure 2 Viseu, Portugal.

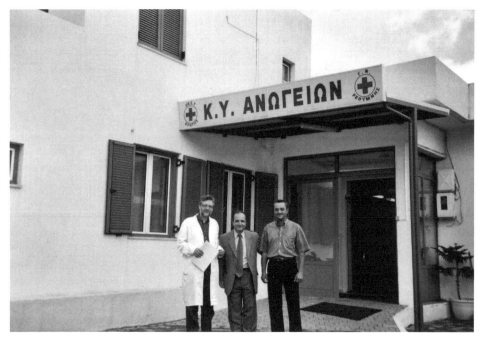

Figure 3 Anogia, Greece.

Figures 1–3 Extended general practice (Finland, Portugal, Greece). The scale of the buildings at Kangasala, Viseu and Anogia indicates the increased size and scope of the modern extended general practice. The picture of the Viseu Health Centre shows Dr Andrea Wild, one of the IPC researchers, standing between the senior community nurse and social assistant at the centre. Three of the Cretan general medical practitioners feature in the photograph at Anogia.

Future prospects

In the first book to be published as a result of the international research programme from which our four case exemplars are drawn, we defined six key relationships for health professions. These are:

- within their own profession
- with other professions
- with policy makers
- with new partners
- with the public
- with patients.[11]

In the twenty-first century all are of paramount significance and the earlier text examines how each relationship now requires its own complex of supporting values and resources. In the twentieth century, arguably, the situation was somewhat simpler and the same could only be said for a profession's internal relationships and its members' individual encounters with patients.

The new sixfold framework offers a useful starting point for understanding the contribution of the extended general practice and its organisational counterparts in modern primary care development to overall social as well as economic capital. An understanding of their relational value and potential points the way towards an assessment of future prospects, for each of the six models described in this book.

The extended general practice scores well across the board, but particularly in terms of individual patients and collaborative interprofessional developments. But there are deficits, as the experience at Viseu and Anogia in particular illustrate. While resource-rich Kangasala and Wimborne have successfully delivered on policy and new partnerships, the shift of general practice towards being a modern, complex organisation has required a level of management which elsewhere has not been sufficient to avoid, for example, professional divisions in Portugal and policy implementation failures in Greece. And both Viseu and Anogia are, it should be remembered, national exemplar sites. Moreover, even within the profession of family medicine itself, the growing gradation of new roles at all locations has the potential at least to reduce the solidarity of past peer-based relationships. General practice is no longer a single set of roles but rather a philosophy within which a growing number of occupations can operate.

Prospectively it can be better for this change, although in some cases allied health professionals may have to swallow hard before they accept the nomenclature of general practice. Overzealous retention of rights to autonomy by family doctors can put at risk the extension of general practice. And as we shall see in the chapters that follow, a number of countries have decided that the GP is either too expensive or protectionist (e.g. China, Croatia, Tanzania) to be the basis of their attempts at primary care-oriented systems development. Several have opted for alternative 'community practitioners' instead. But from the perspective of the individual and his or her desire to have a personal physician, this is clearly a pity. Moreover, recent European research suggests that traditional individual relationships can be successfully translated to tomorrow's extended practice teams,[12] and thence to wider public health responsibilities and functions.

Conceptually, the extended general practice should be a source of substantial and sustained social capital. For those concerned that the combination of scientific medicine and electronic communications might overwhelm relationships-based healthcare, it is important that extended general practice should succeed. Its advance, from this viewpoint, is needed at least as much in developing countries as it is in those states where it is already established. But there is a risk and there are reservations. Suppose, instead of Kangasala, Viseu, Anogia and Wimborne, this chapter had described defensive small or single-handed street corner surgeries. Not only do they still exist, in many places they are actually on the increase: bastions of independent and often private general medical practice with minimal public or other professional contributions. Participation in external policy developments and partnerships does not happen here and, as we shall see in our examples from Sydney (*see* p.70) and South Africa (*see* p.85), alternative service approaches to primary care can all too easily overtake the self-interested general practice. A spirit of real generosity is required alongside generalism for the prospects of the extended model to remain positive. The pressures of public accountability are rightly proving hard to resist and the dangers of the demise of general practice should not be under-estimated.

References

1 Meads G, Ashcroft J (2000) *Relationships in the NHS*. London: RSM Press.
2 Ritsatakis A, Barnes R, Dekker E et al. (2000) *Exploring Policy Development in Europe*. Copenhagen: WHO.
3 Santana P (2002) Poverty, social exclusion and health in Portugal. *Social Science and Medicine*. **55**: 333–45.
4 Sissouras A, Souliotis K (eds) (2003) *Health, Health Care and Welfare in Greece*. Athens: Hellenic Republic Ministry of Health and Welfare.
5 Tountas Y, Karnaki P, Pavi E (2002) Reforming the reform: the Greek national health system in transition. *Health Policy*. **62**: 15–29.
6 NHS Executive (1994) *Letter 79. Developing NHS purchasing and GP fundholding*. Leeds: DoH.
7 Meads G (ed.) (1996) *A Primary Care-led NHS. Putting it into practice*. London: Churchill Livingstone.
8 Department of Health (2004) *Investing in General Practice. The New General Medical Services Contract*. London: DoH.
9 Campbell S, Roland M (2005) The experience of the United Kingdom. In: Garcia-Peña C, Munoz O, Duran L et al. (eds) *Family Medicine at the Dawn of the 21st Century*. Cuauhtémoc: Instituto Mexicano de Seguro Salud.
10 NHS Alliance (2005) *So You Thought You Knew All About NHS Primary Care*. National Primary and Care Trust Development Programme. CANDO Series. Retford: NHS Alliance.
11 Meads G, Ashcroft J (2005) *The Case for Interprofessional Collaboration in Health and Social Care*. Oxford: Blackwell Science.
12 Wensing M, Mainz J, Ferreira P et al. (1998) General practice care and patients' priorities in Europe: an international comparison. *Health Policy*. **45**: 175–86.

Country profile sources

Finland, Portugal and Greece

a Population Division of the Department of Economic and Social Affairs of the United Nations Secretariat (2005) World Population Prospects: The 2004 Revision Population Database. http://esa.un.org/unpp/ (accessed 22/06/05).
b Central Intelligence Agency (2005) The World Factbook. www.cia.gov (accessed 27/06/05).
c World Health Organization (2005) Core Health Indicators, WHO Statistical Information System. www.who.int (accessed 23/06/05).
d Adapted from World Health Organization (2005) WHO mortality database. www.who.int (accessed 08/09/05).
e World Health Organization (2005) World Health Statistics 2005, WHO Statistical Information System. www.who.int (accessed 23/06/05).
f European Observatory on Health Systems and Policies (2002) Health Care Systems in Transition HiT summary Finland. www.euro.who.int/observatory (accessed 23/07/05).

g European Observatory on Health Systems and Policies (2004) Health Care Systems in Transition HiT summary Portugal. www.euro.who.int/observatory (accessed 24/08/05).

h World Health Organization (1996) Regional Office for Europe Copenhagen. Health care systems in transition: Greece. www.who.dk (accessed 25/08/05).

i World Health Organization (1998) Regional Office for Europe. Highlights on health in Greece. www.who.dk (accessed 25/08/05).

England

a Adapted from Office for National Statistics (2005) T 04: England; estimated resident population by single year of age and sex; mid-2004 population estimates. London: Office for National Statistics. www.statistics.gov.uk (accessed 26/08/05).

b Adapted from Office for National Statistics (2001) *Census 2001: national report for England and Wales*, p.121. London: Office for National Statistics.

c World Health Organization (2005) United Kingdom, 2005. www.who.int (accessed 23/06/05).

d Adapted from Office for National Statistics. *UK Business: activity, size and location – 2004*, Statistical Framework Division, Table A2.1. www.statistics.gov.uk (accessed 08/09/05).

e National Statistics (2005) *Population Trends*. **120**: 54.

f Adapted from Office for National Statistics. *Mortality statistics cause: review of the Registrar General on deaths by cause, sex and age, in England and Wales, 2003*; DH2: 30. London: Office for National Statistics. www.statistics.gov.uk (accessed 26/08/05).

g Adapted from the Department of Health (2004) All staff in the NHS: 1994 to 2004, data as at 30 September 2004. www.dh.gov.uk/workforcestatistics (accessed 14/09/05).

h Department of Health (2005) *Forward Plan 2005–2006*. London: DoH.

i Department of Health (2002) *Improvement, Expansion and Reform: the next 3 years' Priorities and Planning Framework 2003–2006*. London: DoH.

Chapter 4

The managed care enterprise

Introduction

The managed care enterprise is most definitely on the move. With powerful sponsors, especially in the pharmaceutical industry, its rapid development is a contemporary global phenomenon. Just as in the last chapter we cited modern primary care organisations in the UK championing the cause of Relational Health Care through extended general practices, so too it would be easy now to find as many advocates among the same fraternity of the managed care enterprise. Indeed, the latter figures rather more prominently in, for example, the NHS Director of Primary Care's recent national Progress Report,[1] with frequent references to primary care trusts that have adopted and adapted managed care protocols and procedures from the likes of EverCare and the Kaiser Permanente Foundation in the US. At times it can seem that the movement towards managed care is irresistible, not least as we have noted in developing countries where resource shortages are such that donor dependency on the West has been virtually absolute (*see* pp.1–6).

It is important therefore from a primary care perspective to understand the changes as an opportunity rather than a threat. The new enterprise is as much about the management by those in primary care of their whole health environment as it is about the management of primary care itself. To both tasks it brings skills and resources that were previously unavailable, especially in terms of the use of computers to take forward both quality and knowledge management on the patient's behalf. Managed care should always bring shorter waiting times, better access, fewer wrong diagnoses and prescriptions, and more effective prevention techniques and screening programmes. It can genuinely empower both professionals and patients and, indeed, it is not unreasonable to regard the standards of managed care as a modern entitlement.

But it also brings fixed budgets, a scale of priorities for different clinical conditions and their interventions, and external controls. Managed care enterprises compete, and they compete on cost. Their performance is monitored in public by politicians. Some primary care professionals will play a leading role in their organisational innovations, but many others are alienated. Moreover, managed care enterprises also attract investment from and returns for parties and partners who previously played no part in health systems, and for whom primary care is not their core business. The issue of cultural fit, as we shall see from our four case exemplars below, is crucial. The imposition of the managed care enterprise, as the experience of parts of Canada illustrates, can produce unexpected failures, just as the Thai and Mexican developments, grounded in their local context, seem surprising successes. Nevertheless, internationally, the managed care enterprise is the modern primary care organisation that most represents globalisation. It is here to stay.

Puebla

A primary healthcare clinic on the side of a volcano with hand-made 'Emergency' warning notices and treacherous unmade roads is not normally where you would expect to find a private sector health insurance company. But the reach of the US-sponsored managed care movement is long and, after all, Mexico is a neighbour of the US and, with Canada, part of a formal North American trading alliance. In Puebla, one of the poorest of Mexico's 31 states, an organisational model with its roots in Californian health maintenance and New England life sciences organisations is an example of this international exchange, in both monetary and moral currencies.

At Puebla each clinic serves around 2500 people. Twenty clinics form a zone for supervision and audit purposes. These management responsibilities reside with the *Oportunidades* branch of the main Mexican health insurance company, the *Instituto Mexicano del Seguro Social* (IMSS). Notwithstanding its independent status, IMSS is a treasured national institution that transcends political change at governmental level. It provides healthcare coverage for over 56 million people, more than half the country's total population. In addition to health insurance and health management, its portfolio includes pensions, disability and unemployment benefits, and food aid. Employee contributions are its chief source of income, with the *Oportunidades* scheme also attracting not only central government funds but World Bank awards as well. As a managed care enterprise its principal counterparts and competitors are either the municipal insurance programmes which now operate in around 40% of Mexico's states, or the Ministry of Health's own Popular Insurance scheme which offers 78 interventions nationally to more than 31 million people.

Market share changes. The national *Progresa* project for indigenous groups, for example, has been largely subsumed into the facilities of the *Oportunidades* management since 2001. The post-millennium arrival of a centre right coalition central government with a reform agenda based on the extension of both primary care and private enterprise has favoured the IMSS managed care philosophy. One in 25 of its employees are engaged in audit activities. Substitution and secondary care controls are key features of the IMSS regime. At Puebla the lead professional in each clinic is a qualified and experienced community nurse. She is the only permanent appointment and delivers a minimum package of 14 healthcare programmes each approved by condition-specific National Institutes for evidence-based clinical quality in Mexico City (19 in all). These programmes address, for example, the public health priorities of diarrhoea, respiratory diseases, tuberculosis and reproductive health.

The IMSS Marginalization Index is used to determine local allocations. Nationally IMSS contracts for 20 000 year six trainee doctors for 12-month community service periods attached to the *Oportunidades* clinics. Here they provide medical back-up to the nurses with radio communication links to 40 IMSS hospitals. The nurses are under the state-level clinical supervision of a peripatetic IMSS principal nursing officer. Together with the Popular Insurance scheme, IMSS offers a total of 108 health interventions with their designated pharmacare options, the additional items being available for either individual purchase or state- and municipal-level commissioning. It is a growth business. Today's patients in Puebla are tomorrow's premium payers.

High up in the Puebla mountains such agendas are not apparent. The clinic thrives. It is especially well used by the local women, two of whom have been trained as a health promoter and maternity aid. The local men, under their influence, have constructed an additional consulting room and a latrine at the clinic, which now hosts some of the local traditional healers as well. There is a community management group, with its members identified against the management's individual health programmes. They effectively market the services of IMSS *Oportunidades* and have successfully petitioned the state authorities to set up two more IMSS-managed clinics in nearby rural neighbourhoods. Each of these provides not just a clinical centre but a focus for economic development through the exchange of produce and the development of local support and educational services.

Over 1000 new clinics have been built in Mexico since the 2001 reforms for decentralisation commenced, with the number belonging to IMSS rising to around 4000. Here in Puebla the extended general practice is not an option, but surprisingly, given the American affluence of its origins, the managed care enterprise, operating competitively to protocols and premiums, is. Mexico has 78 000 doctors in all. Only 3% are fully qualified general medical practitioners, and they practise mostly in private practice in the larger cities. For the majority of the poorer parts of the world the modern primary organisation has to move on beyond the GP. In Mexico, as IMSS continually demonstrates, this means the management of the care enterprises include the identifying and disseminating of appropriate service models from any appropriate source, anywhere and everywhere.[*]

Mexico	
1 Capital city:	Mexico City
2 Demographic factors:	
Population size (million)[a]	107.03 (2005)
Age profile[a]	10.1% (aged < 5), 5.3% (aged 65 and over) (2005)
Ethnicity[b]	Mestizo (Amerindian-Spanish) 60%; Amerindian or predominantly Amerindian 30%; white 9%; other 1%

[*] IMSS in fact over 2004–2005 identified nine countries as relevant to its particular development needs and compiled contributions from these in a single text for use by its members.[2]

3 Socioeconomic factors:
GDP per capita (International $)[c] 8979 (2002)
Health expenditure per capita
(International $)[c]   550 (2002)
Health expenditure per GDP[c]   6.1% (2002)
Main industry[b]   Food and beverages; tobacco;
                                       chemicals; iron and steel; petro-
                                       leum; mining; textiles; clothing;
                                       motor vehicles; consumer durables;
                                       tourism

4 Health factors:
Life expectancy at birth[c]   74.0 (M 72.0/F 77.0) (2003)
Five main causes of death
(rate per 100 000 population)[d]   Diseases of circulatory system,
                                       98.74; external causes, 85.56;
                                       endocrine, nutritional and meta-
                                       bolic diseases, 62.58; neoplasms,
                                       58.40; diseases of digestive system,
                                       42.52 (2001, ICD 10 used, coverage
                                       rate 96.0%)

5 Organisational factors:
Primary care model   IMSS (*Instituto Mexicano del Seguro
                                       Social*) and Mexican Ministry of
                                       Health, SSA (*Secretaría de Salud*),
                                       health centres and stations, hospital
                                       rooms; unofficial '*micro empresas*' in
                                       rural and remote areas; traditional
                                       medicine for indigenous peoples
Resources (health personnel)[e]   17.1 physicians/10 000 pop. (2001);
                                       10.8 nurses and midwives/10 000
                                       pop. (1999)
Financing[f,g]   Mexican Social Security Institute
                                       IMSS (federal budget, contributions
                                       from employees and employers in
                                       private sector); insurance scheme
                                       for state workers by ISSSTE (*Instituto
                                       de Seguridad y Servicios Sociales de los
                                       Trabajadores del Estado*) (federal/state
                                       budgets; employees contribution);
                                       petroleum company PEMEX funds;
                                       federal budget for the Armed Forces
                                       (SEDENA); Popular Health
                                       Insurance '*Oportunidades*' by SSA for
                                       self-employed or unemployed;
                                       federal block grants/supplemental
                                       funds (to municipalities); out-of-

| | pocket payments; private health insurance funds; external loans |
| Lead primary care practitioners | Trainee doctors, community nurses and traditional healers |

Policy priorities

A *Choice, coverage, and equitable access to healthcare*
A package of up to 105 services including all drugs via Popular Health Insurance *'Oportunidades'·* a basic package of 13 priority programmes (preventive/promotion focused) defined at National Health Council and implemented at state level

B *Financing*
Promoting new funding for local state level, including out-of-pocket payments and membership fees

C *Restructure insurance programmes*
Incorporating *Progresa* programme (*Oportunidades Sedesol*) for the poor (including primary healthcare) into the government-led Popular Health Insurance programme

D *Social marketing*
National crusade for quality of care

E *Decentralisation, partnerships and participation*
Promoting social participation in service management at health centres; effective coordination of different levels of care sector; local participation in priority setting through nationwide network of healthy municipalities and multisectoral health promotion; healthy schools about improved lifestyles

F *Management and regulation*
Establishment of national quality standards for local- and state-level committees; incentive mechanisms for communities involved in health-care and education as well as generating resources; evidence-based medicine with a National Institute; shifting population towards using more primary healthcare services

G *Human resources management and development*
Incentive mechanisms encouraging doctors in family medicine; new training programmes for managers at all levels and for health promoters, nationwide education programmes to improve performance of community committees

Auckland

Despite its small population of just over four million, New Zealand was our first port of call for research in 2003 because its modernisation processes were the most easily identifiable with the development of new primary care organisations. In Auckland, alongside the Pegasus Group, the Pro-Care Independent Practice Association (IPA) has epitomised this development, which, in 2005, is being disseminated nationwide by the coalition government that was elected in parallel with that of New Labour in the UK in 1997 and 2001. Their political agendas are strikingly similar, with New Zealand launching its own national health plans in December 2000 and new Primary Health Care Strategy in February 2001. These coincided with a new ten-year plan for the NHS and the arrival of primary care trusts in England.

The Auckland primary health organisations are a hybrid model which reflect New Zealand's different cultural characteristics combining, on the one hand, a commitment to protect the needs of such indigenous peoples as the Maoris and South Sea Islanders that dates back to the Treaty of Waitangi in 1840 and, on the other, an equal determination to defend the medical health professional's right to manage his own practice. The New Zealand managed care enterprise looks to release a spirit of entrepreneurialism in the public interest. Although technically not-for-profit, it has also been seen as a means of allowing public funds to accumulate in private reserves.[3] The post-2001 strategy has sought to address this concern. Government officials asserted to us at interview that:

> *Primary health organisations will be combinations of multiprofessional providers working with local communities to improve health and to reduce inequalities. We are moving to a system where services are coordinated around the needs of a defined group of people.*

But this needs-led philosophy has not meant more national prescription in terms of organisational developments and innovations in primary care, resulting in both greater diversity and differences.

Accordingly, in Auckland, our interviewees' responses reflected a continuing dichotomy of perspectives. Pro-Care is still led and controlled by its 370 general medical practitioners. Since the Gibbs Report recommending the separation of purchasing and providing responsibilities and the subsequent 1993 Health and Disabilities Act,[4] these GPs have become fully absorbed into the managed care enterprise. On the one hand, as individual medical providers they are in a position to take advantage of a heady mix of funding sources. Co-payments are standard and two-thirds of the income for an IPA member retaining private independent status may come from patients or their representatives' fees for service. But in return they must comply with Pro-Care's management of national good practice guidelines, offer a limited range of designated care services and comply with the national Ombudsman's quality standards.

These commissioning functions are also led and controlled by general medical practitioners within the Pro-Care Group who appoint their own chief executive and have their own shareholders board. For more than a decade these functions have progressively increased via the allocations received through the country's 22 district health boards from the national funding authority in Wellington. In this guise, GP interviewees spoke passionately of their commitment to community, to minorities and to New Zealand itself. The country is distinctive among countries with primary managed care enterprises in its use of the model of the managed care enterprise for service growth rather than rationalisation, underpinned by new clinical guidelines.[5]

With this ethos, too, new primary-based purchaser-providers have competed for both public opinion and profit with autonomous hospital-based Crown Health Enterprises as well as other Independent Practice Associations. At the neighbouring Pegasus Group the drive for both cost and clinical effectiveness has led to mergers and management restructuring with a range of pharmacists, nurses and other independent family health services professionals being taken into the new primary health organisation. It has also led to a growing diversity of commissioned services through contracts with both local charitable and commercial agencies, as the Pegasus governance model has increasingly incorporated community groups and representatives.

At Pro-Care, risk analysis remains all important. Its protocols and procedures weigh the balance of opportunities and threats arising, especially for general medical practitioners, from a managed care regime that brings together the performance requirements of the national government's annual Statement of Objectives on the one hand with practice business plans on the other. And the district health board has the power to pull the plug if, for example, budgetary and hospital waiting time (four months) targets are not met. They can go elsewhere. Given internal competition within Pro-Care and the presence of Pegasus they could even go elsewhere within an existing primary health organisation. Whether leading or not, Auckland is the managed care enterprise at the edge in today's international health systems environment.

By the end of 2004 there were 20-plus new multiprofessional primary health organisations operating alongside IPAs across New Zealand. Central direction on structural form and status remained minimal. This degree of licence caused concerns in relation to both equity and efficiency issues, notwithstanding progress towards national funding formulae based on public health data rather than secondary care referrals. Curiously, we found these concerns at the most acute among the non-governmental agencies which, in policy terms, have been targeted for their potential in terms of resource partnerships. At Rotorua, for example, the staff of the Tipu Ora Trust for community health development expressed their fears of primary health organisations becoming 'burgeoning bureaucracies' in response to the range of their new roles and responsibilities. The Trust has decided itself to preserve its voluntary spirit as a wellbeing programme with a spiritual attachment to its homeland, and not to either join or become a new primary health organisation itself. Another NGO, the Plunket Society, has reacted to what it sees as the growing dangers of excessive organisational diversity in primary health services by enforcing new nationwide standards for all its care workers.

Nevertheless, without formally placing secondary care contracts as a comprehensive responsibility of its primary health personnel, in Auckland the mix of managed care enterprises has produced what one Pro-Care director called 'the necessary grit in the system'. The patients who enrol with Pro-Care receive community service cards. These give them access to an ever-increasing range of healthcare facilities: some from the organisation's own medical professionals; some from their subcontractors and subordinates; and even some from those commissioned from Pegasus or Plunket. New Zealand is certainly not neat and tidy in its development of the managed care enterprise, but it is unequivocally novel.

New Zealand

1 Capital city: Wellington

2 Demographic factors:
  Population size (million)[a]   4.03 (2005)
  Age profile[a]   6.8% (aged < 5), 12.3% (aged 65
                                                    and over) (2005)
  Ethnicity[b]   New Zealand European 74.5%;
                                                    Maori 9.7%; other European 4.6%;
                                                    Pacific Islander 3.8%; Asian and
                                                    others 7.4%

3 Socioeconomic factors:
  GDP per capita (International $)[c] 21 943 (2002)
  Health expenditure per capita
  (International $)[c]   1857 (2002)
  Health expenditure per GDP[c]   8.5% (2002)
  Main industry[b]   Food processing; wood and paper
                                                    products; textiles; machinery; trans-
                                                    portation equipment; banking and
                                                    insurance; tourism

4 Health factors:
  Life expectancy at birth[c]   79.0 (M 77.0/F 82 .0) (2003)
  Five main causes of death
  (rate per 100 000 population)[d]   Diseases of circulatory system,
                                                    283.06; neoplasms, 201.44; external
                                                    causes, 69.11; diseases of respiratory
                                                    system, 53.22; endocrine, nutri-
                                                    tional and metabolic diseases, 26.10
                                                    (2000, ICD 10 used, coverage rate
                                                    99.4%)

5 Organisational factors:
  Primary care model   District Health Boards fund Primary
                                                    Health Organisations (PHOs) as
                                                    contracted not-for-profit networks,
                                                    including a wide range of public and
                                                    private agencies; Independent
                                                    Practice Associations (IPAs) as
                                                    'managing agents' of GP collabora-
                                                    tives with community health
                                                    budgets
  Resources (health personnel)[e]   22.3 physicians/10 000 pop. (2001);
                                                    90.3 nurses and midwives/10 000
                                                    pop. (2003)

Financing[h]	General taxation; Accident Insurance Scheme funds; out-of-pocket payments; voluntary private health insurance funds
Lead primary care practitioners	GPs

Policy priorities
A *Equitable access to healthcare*
  Promoting equity in healthcare (e.g. targeted funding formula and provision of services based on health needs, and financial and geographical deprivation, including Maori populations)
B *Decentralisation and participation*
  District Health Boards coordinate local development programmes; promotion of public involvement within the governance of PHOs
C *Management*
  Improvement through initiatives to improve standards of care via continuous quality improvement; capitation-based funding through registering patients

Calgary

Canada. Oh Canada! So desperate to be different. So keen to impress. So many people at every meeting we attended, often all talking at once. So many versions of the Canadian health system on offer and all beautifully written up by excellent academics in first class universities. But not one constituting the heart of a whole health system. Interview schedules designed for ones and twos held in board rooms with committees as respondents. Most bizarre of all, a government-recommended 3000 kilometre flight from Ottawa to the 'best' Canadian primary care organisation, notwithstanding Ontario's (and Quebec's) much-vaunted *Centres Locaux de Services Communitaires* on the doorstep.[6,7] And, of course, above all else, the desire to be distinctly different from those south of the border. And yet, when we arrived at Calgary, it was unequivocally the North American model of the managed care enterprise that we encountered, albeit with a Canadian facade. Calgary, after all, is a city where previous researchers found that programme budgets reflected positional professional power and activity levels as much as local population needs.[8]

The façade is that of universal access to fully comprehensive healthcare under the terms of the 1984 Canada Health Act. The Medicare national health insurance scheme with its requirement of portability of benefits across Canada's ten provinces and two territories is popularly regarded as a national treasure, an important historic legacy of a geographically huge country keen to preserve those pioneering developments that can give 30 million people a sense of common kinship and identity. In the health region of Calgary, within the province of Alberta, the medical director with responsibility for community services regarded such a perception as mere rhetoric, at least in relation to primary care: 'the orphaned child' of Health Canada.

Canada is a country where, in many areas, half of the population do not have automatic registered access to a general medical practitioner; where Physicians' Networks have resisted the central government's past preference for interprofessional Family Health Networks; where nine out of ten doctors retain private practitioner status and often decline to see the patients of community health centres; and where personal or occupational insurance is required to cover the costs of standard prescriptions and urgent drugs purchases to which Medicare provides only limited access. Even the integrated care pilots at community health centres for older people have the preservation of autonomy as their main principle, with family medicine viewed as a point of entry to an integrated service rather than its central constituent.[9]

In the Calgary Health Region this context and the local commitment to modernising primary care has given rise to a distinctive 'social marketing' approach. With its presentational emphasis, this is the culturally acceptable face of primary managed care characterised by a language of 'connectivity', 'community development' and optimal 'affiliation'. The softness of these words is not in any way a deceit. The commitment to a consumerist model based on the needs of those least able to pay is indisputably authentic, but it should not disguise the fundamentally market-oriented mindset.

So the management of the Calgary Health Region (CHR) operate entrepreneurially as a modern network-based organisation dedicated to delivering performance and best value through diversity. Accordingly, their 'care score card' turns objectives for health promotion and healthcare improvement into annual, three- and five-year business targets at the Eighth and Eighth Health Unit in the city centre; into the terms of contract for a single-handed GP at the Midpark Way Clinic keen to obtain CHR funding for an electronic laboratory; and into the referral protocols to a new Diagnostic and Treatment Centre from the physicians' own out-of-hours service. This is targetry applied to stakeholding with a sophistry and sophistication for which we found no rival anywhere else on earth. Absolutely critical to this management of disparate interests and multiple primary care service outlets is the creation and control of a credible, consistent and comprehensive regionwide information system. Termed Calgary Health Link (CHL), directed by a consultant paediatrician, with the Salvation Army and United Way charities among its high profile sponsors, with global research partnerships for clinical protocol and software development and the main local telephone company (Telus) responsible for its original start-up grant, CHL is all things to all people. Most important, it is seen as both the voice of the consumer and the agent of the professional, whatever their employment status.

The social marketing is of 'deliberative decision making' across the region so that 'appropriate care is by the appropriate provider' – in the words of both CHL and the region's executive director for primary care development. The latter is a nurse, and in practice, many nurses are now managing and providing the frontline services in Calgary. Substitution for doctors and for past omissions is an important if implicit theme of this managed care enterprise, as it is of many counterparts around the world. Historically this is a country that has been relatively weak in its intermediate executive tiers and functions. Canada-wide, the Calgary Health Region is part of the modernising reforms in favour of primary care, which have been triggered by a crisis of public confidence in Medicare.

This culminated in large-scale hospital bed reductions, major provincial over-spends and illicit local charging policies in many parts of the country by 1999–2000.[10] The crisis led, under Saskatchewan's political leadership, to the 2002 Romanow Commission report on *The Future of Health Care in Canada* and a subsequent $16 billion transfer fund from Ottawa designed to not only promote modern quality and diversity in primary care but also to restore the core Canadian values of Medicare across the country.

With the proportion of GDP on healthcare threatening to escalate into the 14–16% bracket, which is now the norm in the states south of the Canadian border, Canadian policy makers had to find ways not just of publicising more effectively the primary care values of prevention, continuity and empower-ment, but also generating real efficiencies by incentivising different providers to integrate their interventions in favour of earlier detection, evidence-based outcomes and home care. While still championing choice and freedom, Canadian style. Toronto's 28 multiprofessional partnership *Centres Locaux de Services Communitaires* offered a valuable service role model. Their compulsory outreach requirements and mixed sponsorship mechanisms can involve more than 50 funders for a single health centre in one locality, such as Carlton on the outskirts of Ottawa. This means youth and community workers are employed alongside doctors, nurses and alternative therapists in staff groups of 50–100 operating in catchment areas of up to half a million people. Many of these will have alternative payment plans and private insurance options – which in the Calgary Health Region now offer simply another source of support for the overall health system and another seat or two on the governing boards for primary care. At a community health centre this now comprises 15-plus members.

Nationwide the transfer fund produced 140 CHR-type projects in its first year. By early 2004, when we met them, the provincial directors of primary care – mostly nurses – were actually having to meet monthly to disseminate the learn-ing and develop together. Remote and electronic communications were not enough. The managed care enterprise in Canada, as elsewhere, has a real momentum not least because around a third of its resources and direction come from individual payers themselves. New national Ombudsman powers have been required, provincial regulatory requirements have been tightened; even general medical practitioners have felt compelled to join corporately into provincial groupings. As Canada is discovering, the managed care enterprise is not a free market vehicle, whatever its origins. As a new primary care agency it belongs very much to the category of new and complex learning organisations with all the unsolved mystery this entails.

Canada

1 Capital city: Ottawa

2 Demographic factors:
   Population size (million)[a]   32.27 (2005)
   Age profile[a]   5.3% (aged < 5), 13.1% (aged 65
                                                     and over) (2005)
   Ethnicity[b]   British Isles origin 28%; French
                                                     origin 23%; other European 15%;
                                                     Amerindian 2%; other, mostly
                                                     Asian, African, Arab 6%; mixed
                                                     background 26%

3 Socioeconomic factors:
   GDP per capita (International $)[c] 30 429 (2002)
   Health expenditure per capita
   (International $)[c]   2931 (2002)
   Health expenditure per GDP[c]   9.6% (2002)
   Main industry[b]   Transportation equipment; chemi-
                                                     cals; minerals; food products; wood
                                                     and paper products; fish products;
                                                     petroleum; natural gas

4 Health factors:
   Life expectancy at birth[c]   80.0 (M 78.0/F 82.0) (2003)
   Five main causes of death
   (rate per 100 000 population)[d]   Diseases of circulatory system,
                                                     248.21; neoplasms, 208.21; external
                                                     causes, 71.47; diseases of respiratory
                                                     system, 57.63; diseases of nervous
                                                     system, the eye and adnexa, and the
                                                     ear and mastoid process, 30.97
                                                     (2000, ICD 10 used, coverage rate
                                                     100.0%)
5 Organisational factors:
   Primary care model   Small, general medical practices,
                                                     multiprofessional Community Health
                                                     Centres (*Centres Locaux de Services
                                                     Communitaires*) and GP-based Family
                                                     Health Networks; hospital teams
                                                     and voluntary services
   Resources (health personnel)[e]   18.9 physicians/10 000 pop. (2002);
                                                     73.5 nurses and midwives/10 000
                                                     pop. (2002)

| Financing[i] | Mainly taxation (majority, federal and provincial) with National health insurance 'Medicare' contributions; federal transfers and block grants for provincial schemes; private health insurance funds; employer-sponsored supplementary benefits for employees (free drugs); out-of-pocket payments; NGO contributions (e.g. 'United Way') |
| Lead primary care practitioners | GPs |

Policy priorities[j]

A *Choice and equitable access to healthcare*
   Improving access to high-quality healthcare for First Nations and Inuit peoples encouraging them to participate in health system; portable 'Medicare' benefits in access to direct outpatient services

B *Primary healthcare and public health*
   Strengthen using new federal block grants, 'Primary Health Care Transfer' aims to provide (re)training programmes for health providers and improve sustainability of health system; smoking control via social marketing and local legislation

C *Partnerships and participation*
   'Public Participation Framework' promotes inclusion of specific health needs (e.g. First Nations) via Advisory Councils and increases popular accountability; promoting 'Resolution Process' between federal and provincial levels to ensure consistency

D *Management*
   Shifting to salaried remuneration of specialists in teaching hospitals and capitation payment for primary healthcare providers from fee-for-service payment; health development exchanges to maximise knowledge management between regions/provinces; strengthen dissemination of evidence-based medicine by Health Canada to regions/provinces

E *Human resources*
   Reintroduction of auxiliary nurses in primary healthcare, especially in marginal areas, where lack of GPs; incorporate family physicians into primary care teams with 'shared care' approach

Ayulthaya

In terms of primary care, does any central policy maker anywhere possess an office as impressive as that of the Permanent Secretary of the Thailand Ministry of Health? His title adorns the modern multistorey building sited amidst manicured lawns, smart walkways and shimmering fountains in a setting on the

outskirts of Bangkok more akin to a theme park than the usual downtown locations occupied by government departments. Given the climate of Thailand, the
term 'blue sky planning' really does seem apposite and while Buddhist shrines
are much in evidence, so too are Disney-style American icons and influence in
Thai plans for future primary care organisations.

   These are termed 'Contracting Units for Primary Care' (CUPC) and are, at
least as a pure paper strategy, indisputably managed care enterprises. As franchises for the provision and purchasing of primary care they are competitive
and market oriented. *Tambons* as municipal authorities; professional clusters
with community support; private clinics approved by the national Medical
Services Department in Bangkok from 2003 to 2004; and, of course, both the
110 private and 800 public hospitals with on-site GP surgeries may each aspire
to local CUPC status. All will charge for their services: 30 Baht (around
50 pence) for anything from a consultation to a surgical procedure, plus top-up
fees for interventions beyond the State's Minimum Health Care Package. This is
now embedded legally in the 2001 National Insurance and 2005 National
Health Security Acts, which built on a prime minister-led national 'Campaign
for Health'. This sought explicitly to promote healthcare both as a universal
right and a commercial opportunity.

   In Thailand, the ethics of Buddhism, business and bureaucracy come together
in a 'new generation' of politics. The CUPC in the ancient sacred city of
Ayulthaya, 100 kilometres north of the capital, captures this combination in its
principles and practice. It is one of six 'Demonstration Dissemination' projects
accredited by the national Health Care Reform Project in Bangkok. This is
advised by the World Bank and academics from Antwerp University and the UK
Royal College of General Practitioners through European Union donor support.
The CUPC is funded through a mixture of charges, charities, 'Sin' tax levies on
tobacco and alcohol sales, and allocations from the per capita formula of the
National Health Security office. This formula is based on the clinically effective
Minimum Health Care Package which is skewed towards ambulatory care,
health promotion and preventive interventions in its calculations for costing
patient episodes (at a total of 1447 Baht per person in 2003 for 46 million
people and extending shortly to include all public service employees).
Moreover, as in Canada, there is also a national primary care transfer fund, but
in this case more New York than Ottawa in its approach. The aim is for the six
health centres serving 60 000 people in Ayulthaya, as elsewhere in Thailand, to
benefit from the income brought in to the country by a targeted one million
medical tourists per annum. From Dubai or Tokyo or Hong Kong to the high-
tech hospitals in central Bangkok and on to the resorts of Phuket and the sandy
southern coastline for rest and recuperation, paying (above the odds) all the
way is the idea, with primary care especially for the poorer parts of the population being the intended beneficiary.

   Like many Thai ideas in Ayulthaya, it remains an aspiration rather than
actual practice. Historically, health service developments in Thailand have been
characterised   by   incremental   opportunism   not   radical   change.[11]
Geographically, the CUPC is administered as a multi-*tambon* province from
offices badly in need not just of physical renovation but of appropriate personnel to perform basic primary care functions. The plan may be for sub-*tambon*
health stations and health centres for every 5000–7000 people, but the reality

is that 30 000 is both the budgetary and the service planning unit, not least for medical manpower. There is only one fully nine-year-qualified family physician and all the local dentists work in private practice. The national model for a CUPC health centre of a four-year-trained professional nurse practitioner with prescribing and dispensing rights, a two-year-trained technical nurse, a public health officer and a dental assistant in one of five teams, all under GP supervision delivering the Minimum Health Care Package, remains elusive, even in such a desirable place as Ayulthaya. The main health centre does have private consulting rooms and a meeting space but it is built next to a temple and it is the religious community not the medical tourists that paid for the facilities.

In 2002–03 there were only 40 000 of these tourists, not one million and while Thai universities now host 26 departments of family medicine and one-third of the country's 30 000 doctors have undertaken general practice conversion courses, over the same period 900 left the public sector for private practice. Moreover, under the influence of the US Medical Colleges, litigation and defensive clinical practice is on the increase, with several of the Thai Medical Councils strongly opposing the shift towards nurse-led care proposed under the terms of CUPC commissioned healthcare packages. The College of Family Physicians is growing but still has less than a thousand members and its representatives described US-based pharmaceutical companies with local partners and production in Thailand as among the principal obstacles to progress in extending primary care.

Managed care and its twin sovereignty of clinical- and cost-effectiveness depends on the integrity and independence of the sources of knowledge. The Ayulthaya CUPC does receive the guidance of the National Health Systems Research Institute, which trawls research evidence and international practice in both clinical service and organisational developments. It is ostensibly independent with its own constitution. But this mirrors that of the country itself in 1997, and the Minister of Health is the Chair of the Institute and overwhelmingly its main financial sponsor. Its staff are 'placed' around many of the country's universities and, of course, its offices in Bangkok are luxuriously located adjacent to those of the Permanent Secretary.

Nevertheless, despite what one WHO representative interviewee described to us as this 'corruption' and fragmentation of the new generation's 'radical' vision by bureaucratic and professional elites, the managed care movement at Ayulthaya is moving on. The CUPC has links to Thammasat University which, with the Thai Nursing Council, has taken direct responsibility for CUPC development in the surrounding villages and remote rural areas which were previously entirely dependent on either private or informal healthcare. As a 'Demonstration Dissemination' site Ayulthaya offers for Thammasat a role model which is projected in ten years to mean comprehensive nurse practitioner provision with back-up five-person general medical practices and 30- to 90-bed community hospitals for 50 000 plus populations. Over half of the people now subscribe to the new services. Teams of nationally approved Inspector Generals are visiting to oversee quality and probity. Thailand's healthcare has historically developed in the past in *ad hoc* ways towards becoming a national system which stretches across its cultural and socioeconomic divisions. In this context the managed care enterprise model is now its modern history.

Thailand

1 Capital city: Bangkok

2 Demographic factors:
  Population size (million)[a]   64.23 (2005)
  Age profile[a]   7.8% (aged < 5), 7.1% (aged 65 and
                                                    over) (2005)
  Ethnicity[b]   Thai 75%; Chinese 14%; other 11%

3 Socioeconomic factors:
  GDP per capita (International $)[c]   7248 (2002)
  Health expenditure per capita
  (International $)[c]   321 (2002)
  Health expenditure per GDP[c]   4.4% (2002)
  Main industry[b]   Tourism; textiles; agricultural
                                                    processing; beverages; tobacco;
                                                    cement; light manufacturing,
                                                    jewellery; electric appliances and
                                                    components; computers; integrated
                                                    circuits; furniture; plastics; tungsten;
                                                    tin production

4 Health factors:
  Life expectancy at birth[c]   70.0 (M 67.0/F 73.0) (2003)
  Five main causes of death
  (rate per 100 000 population)[d]   External causes, 105.75; neoplasms,
                                                    64.80; diseases of circulatory
                                                    system, 53.07; infectious and para-
                                                    sitic diseases, 52.45; diseases of
                                                    respiratory system, 34.63 (2000,
                                                    ICD 10 used, coverage rate 89.1%)

5 Organisational factors:
  Primary care model   'Contracting Units for Primary Care
                                                    (CUPC)' managed local health
                                                    centres; mostly private providers
                                                    plus *tambon* services; new skills-mix
                                                    model (e.g. sanitarians and nurse
                                                    prescribers)
  Resources (health personnel)[e]   3.0 physicians/10 000 pop. (1999);
                                                    16.2 nurses and midwives/10 000
                                                    pop. (1999)
  Financing   General taxation (mainly national);
                                                    out-of-pocket payments; National
                                                    Health Security Scheme funds; 'sin
                                                    tax' (2% tobacco and alcohol, 2003)
  Lead primary care practitioners   Nurses

Policy priorities
A *Universal coverage and public health*
   Through standard package of medical care at *tambon* and sub-*tambon*
   levels; environmental health at *tambons* through block grants
B *Innovative financing*
   Cost control through '30 Baht' payment universal health scheme and
   capitation-funded Contracting Units for Primary Care (CUPC); intro-
   duction of 'sin tax' to support universal health scheme
C *Regulation*
   Peer-based quality assurance for health professionals
D *Participation*
   1997 Constitutional health rights with community participation
   through local administrative organisations
E *Human resources*
   Large-scale fast-track doctor conversion programmes for future family
   physicians; development of continuous education and training for
   health professionals

Future prospects

The economic and executive emphasis of the managed care enterprise would
prima facie suggest that this organisational model of primary care might be the
least conducive to the cause of relational health. Certainly our examples from
Canada and Thailand, in particular, highlight the risks of corporate and
commercial capture alongside continuing professional self-interest. But it

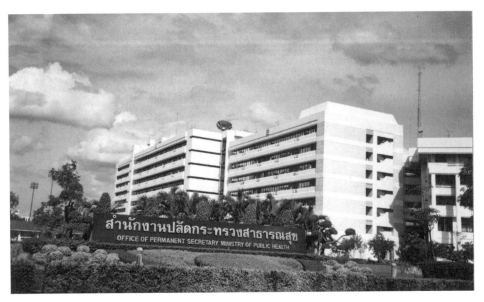

Figure 4   Bangkok, Thailand.

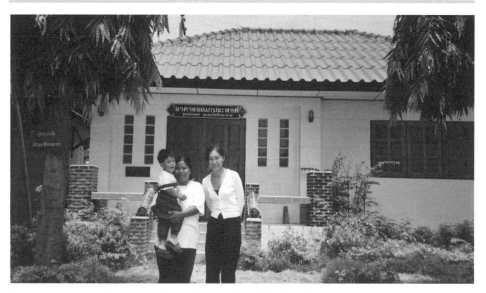

Figure 5   The Managed Care Enterprise, Thailand.

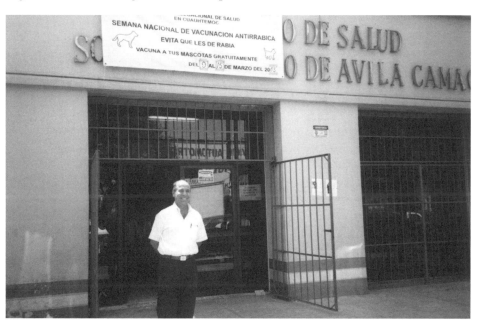

Figure 6   IMSS Clinic, Mexico.

Figures 4–6 The managed care enterprise (Thailand, Thailand, Mexico). The bureaucratic and business sides of managed care are well illustrated in these images from Thailand and Mexico. The office of the senior civil servant in the Ministry of Health in Bangkok is on the grandest scale, while the photograph of Michiyo Iwami and a local woman at the Ayulthaya Health Centre was taken in front of the meeting room used for both health promotion and local Buddhist community meetings. The picture of an IMSS clinic in Mexico illustrates how local primary care complies with national disease management campaigns.

would be wrong to write off the managed care enterprise simply because of its capitalist roots and financial bias. Clearly it is now a culturally compatible innovation in many parts of the world, and the key issue for organisations that champion value for money is how that value is defined: by whom and in whose interests?

Both our case exemplars from New Zealand and Mexico indicate that, where this value is defined in the context of social responsibility and public health stewardship, even by private status companies and professionals, it is tenable for managed care enterprises to significantly enrich health service relationships. While no one profession, other than management itself perhaps, can have the single controlling interest in a multistakeholder-style development, the managed care interest does compel interprofessional contributions to resource efficient integrated care and, as in Ayulthaya, its marketing approach must require a sharper awareness of the paying patient's expressed service requirements as well as trends in public attitudes and clinic attendance.

Policy makers also like the managed care enterprise. Unlike some of its counterparts, it sets out to do what it says it will do. And no more. The dangers of excess expenditure and unanticipated activity volumes are much lower, and anyway the accountabilities for 'overheating' in the system are now at arms length from government residing with autonomous and audited agencies.

But these benefits have to be balanced against the business ethic of managed care. A healthy society is more than a marketplace. The person who presents as a patient is more than a user or a consumer. Purchasing power pays off, in healthcare as with other 'commodities', and the managed care enterprise as the main form of primary care organisation, even for IMSS in Mexico, is untenable when the sociodemographic profile reveals a majority of low-income groups. Here, as elsewhere, the model is divisive and, significantly, in affluent Canada it is not, even in Calgary, the vehicle for universal coverage. In developed countries it can cause considerable public discontent[12] requiring, as in New Zealand, rigorous new complaints management systems.[13] Nevertheless, the managed care enterprise is expanding its scale of operations and its spheres of influence. It will clearly be an important organisational development for primary care throughout the present century. But nowhere should it be the only one.

References

1 Department of Health (2004) *A Responsive and High-quality Local NHS*. London: DoH.
2 Garcia-Peña C, Muñoz O, Duran L et al. (eds) (2005) *Family Medicine at the Dawn of the 21st Century. Themes and arguments*. Mexico City: Instituto Mexicano del Seguro Social.
3 Mays N (2002) Reform and counter reform: how sustainable is New Zealand's latest health system restructuring? *Journal of Health Services Research and Policy*. **7** (supplement): 46–55.
4 Maxwell R (1995) Introduction to the Commonwealth scene. In: Williams R (ed.) *International Developments in Health Care*, pp.3–36. London: Royal College of Physicians.
5 Niessen L, Grijseels E, Rutten F (2000) The evidence-based approach in health policy and health care delivery. *Social Science and Medicine*. **51**: 859–69.
6 Beland F (1999) Preventive and primary care access systems. In: Powell F, Wessen A (eds) *Health Care Systems in Transition*, pp.173–98. London: Sage.

7 Naylor C (1999) Health care in Canada: incrementalism under fiscal duress. *Health Affairs*. **18**(3): 9–26.

8 Mitton C, Donaldson C (2002) Setting priorities in Canadian regional health authorities: a survey of key decision makers. *Health Policy*. **60**: 39–58.

9 Hébert R, Durand P, Dubuc N et al. (2003) PRISMA: a new model of integrated service delivery for the frail older people in Canada. *International Journal of Integrated Care*. Accessed online 18/3/2003.

10 Hughes Tuohy C (2002) The costs and prospects for health care reform in Canada. *Health Affairs*. **21**(3): 32–46.

11 Green A (2000) Reforming the health sector in Thailand: the role of policy actors on the policy stage. *International Journal of Health Planning and Management*. **15**: 39–59.

12 Donelan K, Blendon R, Shoen C et al. (1999) The cost of health system change: public discontent in five nations. *Health Affairs*. **18**(3): 206–16.

13 Paterson R (2002) The patients' complaints system in New Zealand. *Health Affairs*. **21**(3): 70–9.

Country profile sources

Mexico, New Zealand, Canada and Thailand

[a] Population Division of the Department of Economic and Social Affairs of the United Nations Secretariat (2005) World Population Prospects: the 2004 revision population database. http://esa.un.org/unpp/ (accessed 22/06/05).

[b] Central Intelligence Agency (2005) The World Factbook. www.cia.gov (accessed 27/6/05).

[c] World Health Organization (2005) Core Health Indicators, WHO Statistical Information System. www.who.int (accessed 23/07/05).

[d] Adapted from World Health Organization (2005) WHO mortality database. www.who.int (accessed 08/09/05).

[e] World Health Organization (2005) World Health Statistics 2005, WHO Statistical Information System. www.who.int (accessed 23/06/05).

[f] Pan American Health Organization (2002) *Health in the Americas: Mexico*, vol. II. Washington, DC: Pan American Health Organization, pp.379–93.

[g] Pan American Health Organization (2002) *Profile of the Health Services System: Mexico*. Program on Organization and Management of Health Systems and Services. Washington, DC: Pan American Health Organization.

[h] European Observatory on Health Systems and Policies (2002) Health Care Systems in Transition HiT summary New Zealand. www.euro.who.int/observatory (accessed 23/07/05).

[i] Pan American Health Organization (2002) *Health in the Americas: Canada*, vol. II. Washington, DC: Pan American Health Organization, pp.125–140.

[j] Romanow RJ (2002) *Building on Values: the future of health care in Canada – Final report*. Saskatoon: Commission on the Future of Health Care in Canada. Also available online: www.hcsc.gc.ca/english/pdf/romanow/pdfs/HCC_Final_Report.pdf#search ='Building%20on%20Values%3A%20the%20future%20of%20health%20care%20 in%20Canada%20Romanow' (accessed 07/07/05).

Chapter 5

The reformed polyclinic

Introduction

The reformed polyclinic model of primary care seems to be casting off the shackles of its Soviet past. As policy makers have learnt how to devise effective financial and clinical regulatory mechanisms for its controlled development the reformed polyclinic has begun to supply an organisational type which may effectively, given the right circumstances, respond to the twin agenda of public preferences for extended specialist direct access and extended public health improvement performance targets.

While still predominantly associated with Eastern Europe and Central Asia, the reformed polyclinic finds its modern expressions worldwide. Indeed, because the new service model has figured prominently in international health-care reforms during our study period, at the turn of the millennium, our four case exemplars are deliberately drawn from countries well away from the polyclinic's Russian roots. It is characterised now by the controlled incorporation of multiple medical practitioners, including family doctors, into unified intervention programmes, usually at a single site. Each of these retains its separate professional and private status, as a result of which, multiprofessional team-work is usually restricted and wider primary care commissioning activities constrained.

While, as we shall see below, strong governments can effectively shape the development of primary care in polyclinics, as an organisational reform they are essentially a response to modern social market developments in which health professionals' rights to supply-side self-determination remain largely sacrosanct. As such, the number of reformed polyclinic policy initiatives actually continues to expand. Pecuniary benefit allied to specialist standing remains a powerful force for organisational development in primary care.

Singapore

In Singapore the extended general practice meets the managed care enterprise and the outcome since 2001 has been a competitive countrywide system of mixed-status polyclinics subject to state regulation and control. Accordingly, for example, the two family doctors at the neon-lit and shopping mall-sited private Dayspring Medical Clinic are members of the 200-strong General Medical Practitioner Panel, that such new intermediary insurance brokers as the private Parkway Health Foundation can require their premium payers to use prior to any elective hospital referral or admission. On the panel too will be the doctors, GPs or otherwise and often only trainees, who staff the Geyland, Marine Parade and the other seven SingHealth Polyclinics established as independent but Government Linked Companies (GLC) in 2001–02.

At Marine Parade, as at the Dayspring Clinic, specialist services are priced, advertised and staffed (usually from the local private hospitals) according to demand. Since 2001 this has increased markedly for dentistry and declined for physiotherapy. The latter has proved hard to value either clinically or economically, unlike the difference between bed-based or recliner day surgery. The former attracts a higher patient charge in the private clinics, as do 'de luxe' diagnostic facilities and x-ray presentations. Back in the SingHealth GLC establishments, as the number of walk-in callers per day began to exceed 1000 at, for instance, the Geyland Polyclinic we visited during 2003–04, so employers began to augment patient and public contributions with their own direct payments for screening services, occupational health checks and even oral health promotion. Their participation highlights the attraction of the reformed polyclinic through the diversity of the different specialist interests that it can now accommodate.

In Singapore, the melting pot culture means that these interests are very varied indeed with, in healthcare, each aspiring to its own branded provision. In the past this has meant having your own hospital with a special ethos, specialist practitioners and distinctive quality. In Singapore, for example, the Buddhist Chinese Association runs a hospital, as does the Church of the Seventh Day Adventists. Both describe these as public services with a degree of non-selective access. But the price of a secondary care-based first-contact service is high. Even at the General Medicine Clinic of the 400-bed Changi General Hospital, where an open-door policy applies, the initial consultation in 2003–04 costs 80 Singapore dollars. This is ten times the standard level at the SingHealth Polyclinic where pensioners and welfare beneficiaries actually pay a further reduced rate of $4 for the first call.

The lower charges have brought the middle classes into the public service sector, often for the first time. SingHealth practitioners can achieve regular patient lists of 700–800 as family doctors now, while the downward pressure on prices has reduced initial consultation charges in the plethora of specialist and solo private practices to as little as $15. This further extends the take-up of healthcare in a country where house calls are a rarity, prevention has been little practised and, in the words of one of our interviewees who had recently completed his three-year post-qualification GP vocational training, 'the people here have been resigned to disease'. When ill see a specialist, pay or go to the hospital emergency department. This has been the standard sequence.

The government's espousal of the reformed polyclinic model in its post-2001 'Primary Health Care Partnership' is creating a new set of public perspectives as well as compelling changes in provider behaviour. In shifting the profile of private practice to local community settings, it has deployed a battery of state instruments. A national State-run financial holding company ensures preferential investment rates and funding opportunities for the nine SingHealth polyclinics. Their drugs supplies and their patients' prescription charges are heavily subsidised and their services are only available to national identity card holders. New teams of nursing monitors regulate SingHealth practice, which is subject to an ISO standard that exposes the lack of quality control and assurance in private specialist clinics that have traditionally relied on professional peer networks, hospital links and word-of-mouth recommendations for their business and income. They still have to pay full commercial rates and corporate taxes and their commissioning health foundations now have to operate their own separate ambulance services if they want to sustain the private clinic and hospital patient care partnerships.

Many still do. As a result, Singapore is a genuine client-oriented marketplace. The private sector remains sufficiently attractive for many young doctors (and even nurses) to continue to buy themselves out of their post-registration Five-Year Bond of public service so that they can practise independently. But many do not, staying with SingHealth, while those that do leave may well now form or join a polyclinic model of their own, often incorporating traditional medical practitioners to attract a cross-generational demand. In Singapore, modern primary care organisations do not require registered lists or even appointment systems. All they need is paying patients and since 2001 the cross-sectoral developments of reformed polyclinics have demonstrated how to reach as many of these as possible.

Singapore

1 Capital city: Singapore

2 Demographic factors:
   Population size (million)[a]   4.33 (2005)
   Age profile[a]   5.0% (aged < 5), 8.5% (aged 65 and
                                     over) (2005)
   Ethnicity[b]   Chinese 76.7%; Malay 14%; Indian
                                     7.9%; other 1.4%

3 Socioeconomic factors:
   GDP per capita (International $)[c] 25 588 (2002)
   Health expenditure per capita
   (International $)[c]   1105 (2002)
   Health expenditure per GDP[c]   4.3% (2002)
   Main industry[b]   Electronics; chemicals; financial
                                     services; oil drilling equipment;
                                     petroleum refining; rubber process-
                                     ing and rubber products; processed
                                     food and beverages; ship repair;
                                     offshore platform construction; life
                                     sciences

4 Health factors:

Life expectancy at birth[c]	80.0 (M 78.0/F 82 .0) (2003)
Five main causes of death (rate per 100 000 population)[d]	Diseases of the circulatory system, 160.97; neoplasms, 125.78; diseases of the respiratory system, 64.62; external causes, 33.56; endocrine, nutritional and metabolic diseases, 18.23 (2001, ICD 9 BTL used, coverage rate 81.4%)

5 Organisational factors:

Primary care model	Private clinics (80%) and public polyclinics (20%)
Resources (health personnel)[e]	14.0 physicians/10 000 pop. (2001); 44.5 nurses and midwives/10 000 pop. (2003)
Financing[f]	Universal and compulsory employee contributions (6–8% premium of salary) complemented by employer contribution to individual Medical Savings Accounts (MSAs) – for various insurances including Medisave, Medishield (for catastrophic illness) and Eldershield (for disabled); government subsidies for poor and elderly (e.g. Medifund); out-of-pocket payments
Lead primary care practitioners	Specialist physicians

Policy priorities

A *Choice, health promotion and prevention*

Freedom to choose health providers and levels of care; encouraging people to take individual responsibility through unique health financing, and promoting screening and health education at polyclinics

B *Partnerships*

Introduction of 'Managed Healthcare' agencies to stimulate the market aiming at relieving the overuse of public hospitals

C *Regulation*

Introduction of ISO (International Organization for Standardization) 'Quality Healthcare' approach to clinical standards

Copacabana

The capacity of the reformed polyclinic to respond to difference and diversity is more vividly illustrated in Brazil than in any other country today. It is a paradox that an originally communist organisational model for primary care, which was most prevalent before 1990 in the Soviet Union, is now being promoted in a capitalistic Brazil, which has the highest inequalities of income between the rich and the poor on the globe. It was in 1990 that a Brazil still recovering from many years of military dictatorship acquired for the first time, through legislation, the principles of a Unified Health System (SUS). These were: universality, equity, participation, decentralisation and service integration – all underpinned by a first-time commitment to national State funding countrywide, across 5500-plus municipalities.

In the subsequent years the structure has followed. The first building blocks were put in place with the 1993 Basic Operating Rule (BOR), which established a nationwide system of capitation payments to local areas. This was extended through 1998 and 2003 reforms, which established three levels of municipal management, a four-yearly cycle of Popular Health Councils and Regional Health Conferences, and the roll-out of proposals for a minimum of 3000 new primary care centres. Most of these are in modern polyclinic format containing multispecialisms, but what these specialisms are varies hugely depending on the local culture, ethnic profile and economic status.

Copacabana is rich, Western and slick city style. Its new primary care centre is near the railway station, the local park and down the road from the beach: convenient for commuters, children and families, holidaymakers and sunbathers. Heavily guarded and surrounded by railings, its physical profile also reflects local security requirements and crime rates. Its rows of cubicles in which the obstetrician, the gynaecologist, the dermatologist, the paediatrician, the psychiatrist, the geriatrician and all the other specialists provide their sessional inputs, are functional and plain and quickly locked on their occupants' departure. Nobody stays long, neither practitioner nor patient, but the interventions defined and paid for under the terms of the national five-year health plan are proficiently provided and a 10% local health tax even allows the municipality to top up some service levels.

For even in Copacabana the polyclinic is a civic amenity not just a health centre. Elsewhere in Brazil, especially in such new and growing cities as Londrina and São Paulo, are to be found youth workers, drama and occupational therapists, older people's day care and health advocacy groups like the Brave Women's Association of *Jardina Franixcata*. At Copacabana the range is limited to welfare rights advice, drugs misuse counselling and, inevitably, religious representatives from the Roman Catholic Church. The influence of the latter remains pervasive and helps promote, especially among the poorer parts of the population, a sense of obligation in attending the polyclinic for preventive services. Polyclinics have built on this moral mandate in their recruitment across the country of volunteer 'health agents' whose role is that of advocacy, for the disadvantaged patient and, equally, for the polyclinic itself and its wares. This is the polyclinic if not masquerading as a community development agency, then certainly exploiting its strengths. At the time of our fieldwork Brazil was well under way in extending its SUS to 30 million people countrywide.[1]

This success story highlights the beauty of the polyclinic as a modernising public service because it has the twin appeal of direct-access clinical specialisms for the middle classes and aggregated comprehensive healthcare packages for blue-collar workers and those previously disenfranchised from formal healthcare services. For this group it brings the professions to the people, often for the first time, but the selectivity and restriction on a polyclinic's range of interventions means that, even in the Copacabana site's extravagant surroundings of Rio de Janeiro, local people can still supplement their health services through traditional healers on the one hand and private consultants and commercial outlets on the other. Both herbal remedies and cosmetic surgery are on the increase, while every street has its brand named orthodontic clinic and drugs store.

Brazil	
1 Capital city:	Brasilia
2 Demographic factors:	
Population size (million)[a]	186.41 (2005)
Age profile[a]	9.7% (aged < 5), 6.1% (aged 65 and over) (2005)
Ethnicity[b]	White (includes Portuguese, German, Italian, Spanish, Polish) 55%; mixed white and black 38%; black 6%; other (includes Japanese, Arab, Amerindian) 1%
3 Socioeconomic factors:	
GDP per capita (International $)[c]	7762 (2002)
Health expenditure per capita (International $)[c]	611 (2002)
Health expenditure per GDP[c]	7.9% (2002)
Main industry[b]	Textiles; shoes; chemicals; cement; lumber; iron ore; tin; steel; aircraft; motor vehicles and parts; machinery and equipment
4 Health factors:	
Life expectancy at birth[c]	69.0 (M 66.0/F 73.0) (2003)
Five main causes of death (rate per 100,000 population)[d]	Diseases of circulatory system, 151.62; external causes, 100.33; neoplasms, 70.12; diseases of respiratory system, 51.41; endocrine, nutritional and metabolic diseases, 27.51 (2000, ICD 10 used, coverage rate 79.2%)

5 Organisational factors:

Primary care model	Extended multispecialist health and social service centres and historically dominant private sector including traditional medicine
Resources (health personnel)[e]	20.6 physicians/10 000 pop. (2001); 5.2 nurses and midwives/10 000 pop. (2001)
Financing[g,h]	Taxation (federal, state and local) on businesses and social security funds; out-of-pocket payments; voluntary private health insurance funds; external loans
Lead primary care practitioners	Auxiliary nurses and specialist physicians

Policy priorities

A *Universal and comprehensive care through the Unified Health System (SUS)*
  Promotion of universal coverage and equity in healthcare; shifting to integrated care focusing on prevention via family health programme including family medicine with basic community health agents; building joint commitment towards inclusion and pro-poor; promotion of new cross-sectoral national priorities (including nutrition and environmental and epidemiological controls); raising awareness of multiculturalism

B *Decentralisation*
  Consolidating municipality-managed new primary care centres and developing community-owned facilities

C *Partnership and participation*
  Promotion of service – university–community networks; social partici-pation in planning at Health Councils at all levels

D *Human resources*
  Educational programmes focusing on establishing family healthcare teams and prevention at medical universities

Sydney

A polyclinic model may happen by design, as in Singapore and, to a significant extent, Brazil, or by default, as in parts at least of Australia. Central Sydney, especially, is an example of a local health system that has developed in ways that the Area Health Board might not have expected when the Commonwealth government issued its 1998 national strategy for 'General Practice Changing the Future through Partnerships', the stated purpose of which was improved inte-gration.[2] With a 30% increase nationally in the number of qualified general medical practitioners between 1990 and 2000, a Commonwealth-sponsored network of 300 GP professional membership Divisions across Australia and powerful professional leadership, not least at the academic institutions of

Newcastle, Gosford and Sydney in New South Wales, the organisational model for primary care development seemed set to be the extended general practice.

So far it is not so. Certainly there are no central policies that formally support any alternative, but to visit central Sydney is to experience the contemporary polyclinic in its technicoloured reality; not at a single site but as a combination of both competitive and collaborative overlapping service outlets. In reality, the individual professional identity of the GP and position of family medicine are at risk, and being continuously renegotiated.

Take George Street, for example. It runs the one-mile length of the city centre. At the southern tip next to a Murphy's public house is The Rocks, a two-doctor private practice, Dublin style, principally for immigrant Irish residents. Its counterpart is the local Chinese Medical Centre at the downtown end. Between the two lies one of the 570 New South Wales community health centres, with its nurses offering a prescribed range of Commonwealth-approved prevention and screening programmes. But there seem fewer people here, and certainly fewer with nurses than across the road in the Paramount Plaza. In this shopping mall the whole of the mezzanine level is occupied by a commercial service company called 'Primary Health Care'. It is beautifully lit and appointed, with separate reception areas for its physiotherapy, dentistry and medical suites, and excellent pathology and pharmacy facilities. Its literature describes the company's six additional local service outlets in Sydney and its 'partnership' arrangements for referral and exchange with the Chinese Medical Centre and its Oriental linked practices. Those shopping in the Paramount Plaza seem of a different ilk to those going into the less ostentatious premises of the nearby Community Club for a quick meal and work-out plus, if desired, a medical consultation and access to a range of healthy lifestyle aids. And, up at Darling Harbour, there is a third, newer kind of service company model in Harbour Health, with its backroom surgery, sessional doctor and influx of one-off sporting types and tourists. This is located in the midst of the main fashion shops and is clearly community pharmacy-based. Services are essentially over-the-counter and call-in. It is a trendsetter in its own right, as is the cleverly titled Medibank, along the way: a private health insurance company with a reassuringly secure name.

The list of specialist facilities could go on and on. As you get closer to Bondi Beach in Waveney the scope becomes ever more exotic: a combined medical and skin cancer centre; Balance Therapy offering only 'natural medicine'; a New Age health centre; and, of course, a specialist primary care and cosmetic surgery service. And, inevitably, the university and subregional hospitals run their own primary care clinics as well in adjacent neighbourhoods.

Meanwhile in rural New South Wales there is a 20% shortfall in the minimum requirement for GPs. Overall in Australia a quarter of the latter have not joined their professional membership Divisions.[3] Subscription and accreditation remains voluntary. Small towns not so far from Sydney, like Cessnock and Hornsby, have to rely on doctors from China, Afghanistan and elsewhere with three-year work permits. One-third of doctors are in single-handed practices. Another third have two or three practitioners. In the words of one of our interviewees, a member of the Federal Commission on General Practice, 'the registered list is an imposition on the people and an unnecessary assertion of professional power'. A fellow university professor and chair of a GP Division emphasised the Australian principle of 'mateship – giving people a fair go'.

As a result, she saw the emergent Sydney-style polyclinic set-up as 'making use of what is to hand'. What is to hand remains, in the words of executives we interviewed in New South Wales, Medicare, which operates still as 'a specialist billing system' that appears almost as 'hospitalcentric' in its approach and its public perspectives as it was at its inception in 1984. Since 2003 and a further government emphasis on private enterprise and health partnerships, this has become more apparent. Over a long period incremental changes in the Australian healthcare system have been characterised by the conviction that universal coverage and more privately insured practice are not a contradiction.[4] To access Medicare's standard-scale fee payments and heavily subsidised pharmaceutical benefits, each of the George Street clinics described above includes at least one employed or contracted general medical practitioner. Their contribution represents the core funding. The commercial business comes from the effective pricing for top-up sales and supplementary services. At least a third of the monies come direct from patients, or at least from those who can afford to pay. Less than 1% of budgets goes on community mental health services. For all the rich diversity of its polyclinic amenities, Sydney still has its soup runs. The Salvation Army still need to be on patrol in George Street at night.

Australia

1 Capital city: Canberra

2 Demographic factors:
   Population size (million)[a]   20.16 (2005)
   Age profile[a]   6.2% (aged < 5), 12.7% (aged 65
                                              and over) (2005)
   Ethnicity[b]   Caucasian 92%; Asian 7%;
                                              Aboriginal and other 1%

3 Socioeconomic factors:
   GDP per capita (International $)[c] 28 277 (2002)
   Health expenditure per capita
   (International $)[c]   2699 (2002)
   Health expenditure per GDP[c]   9.5% (2002)
   Main industry[b]   Mining; industrial and transporta-
                                              tion equipment; food processing;
                                              chemicals; sports; steel; tourism

4 Health factors:
   Life expectancy at birth[c]   81.0 (M 78.0/F 83.0) (2003)
   Five main causes of death
   (rate per 100 000 population)[d]   Diseases of circulatory system,
                                              255.16; neoplasms, 192.96; external
                                              causes, 65.84; diseases of respiratory
                                              system, 54.72; endocrine, nutritional
                                              and metabolic diseases, 22.32 (2001,
                                              ICD 10 used, coverage rate 100.0%)

5 Organisational factors:

Primary care model[i]	Based on small self-employed GP surgeries, geographic GP Divisions with 100–300 GPs each; skill-mix registered nurses and nurse triage
Resources (health personnel)[e]	24.7 physicians/10 000 pop. (2001); 91.2 nurses and midwives/10 000 pop. (2002)
Financing[i]	General taxation (federal, state and local) and sales tax revenue (10% goods and services tax for state and local governments); mandatory Medicare (national health insurance) contributions (1.5% income tax for wealthy population); out-of-pocket payments; voluntary private health insurance funds
Lead primary care practitioners	GPs and nurses

Policy priorities

A *Health equalities*
  Reducing health inequalities especially among Aboriginal populations
B *Partnerships and participation*
  Positive involvement of private sector through provider competition and development
C *Management and regulation*
  Effective pricing and cost control; development of strategies for effective market management
D *Human resources*
  Development of strategies to combat workforce shortfalls, including foreign recruitment

Santiago

With statutory comprehensive healthcare for workers and their dependants dating back to 1924, Chile has seen itself historically as the leader of Latin America on health systems reform. Its commitment to a national service and to primary care predates that of every country south of Florida. In recent times the raised profile of Cuba and its Health for All policies seem to have served only as a competitive stimulus for the Chilean Ministry of Health to retain this pioneering position. In the South Metropolitan Area of Santiago, for example, the purpose built San Joaquín Health Centre has been, since 2000, one of six initially government-sponsored polyclinic pilots which fulfil this role.

Under the terms of the *Acceso Universal con Garantías Explícitas* (AUGE) national health services programme, the primary care organisation of San

Joaquín offers, through the services of its ten different professionals, both individualised 'family health plans' to its 28 000 locally registered patients and 56 nationally specified interventions for the prevention and cure of specific centrally determined priority conditions. Mental health tops the list of these. The government proposes to both roll out its new organisational model to 28 area health authorities in Chile by 2007 and, at the same time, to progressively transfer their local service management, as in the South Metropolitan patch, to elected zonal mayors and councils.

The aim is to reduce the number of central appointees to the latter from 3000 to 700. The numbers are precise and specific. So too, we were advised at the Ministry in 2003, are the funding formulae for the 85% allocation from the post-1952 National Health Fund: 40% programme budgets and 60% capitation payments with the latter weighted for poverty (up to 18%) and rurality (up to 20%), and the former statistically calculated on projected activity trends and attendance rates. The reformed polyclinic in Santiago is itself a precise and specific strategic development. Hence it is deliberately designed to help accommodate within a local health system modern advanced general medical practice; an incentivised multiprofessional 'team concert'; the controlled contribution of private payers and providers; and enhanced local community and public health developments. Not surprisingly, Chile is a country with an enviable record of preventing 'seepage' in the use of public funds for targeted disadvantaged population groups and their needs.[5]

As a result, San Joaquín is to the reformed polyclinic what Kangasala is to the extended general practice and Auckland's Pegasus Group is to the managed care enterprise. Conceptually, at least, it constitutes modernisation at its most sophisticated. If the Sydney style of polyclinic reflects the ambivalence felt by Australians towards the often-muddled mix of primary care service outlets, there are no such uncertain motives or unintended consequences in Chile. The reformed polyclinic is consciously part of a competitive approach but within firm corporate structures and the cultural constraints of a country that feels it has experienced both benefits and setbacks from past political dictatorships. One of these was responsible in 1981 for establishing, this time as a global pioneer, competitive healthcare purchasing through independent sector but statutory 7% payroll tax-funded *Instituciones de Salud Previsional* (ISAPREs). There are now 14 such health insurance funds with a level of subscribers that has declined from 4 million in 1997 to 2.4 million in 2003. The downward trend reflects the improved performance of their public sector FONASA (National Health Fund) rival; a recognition that the ISAPREs are ill placed to deal with major chronic and communicable diseases;[6] and a continuing market dynamic that dates back at least to the introduction of tendering arrangements in 1968 by the Social Security Ministry for ambulatory care for welfare benefit recipients.

So, in the South Metropolitan Area of Santiago, the San Joaquín polyclinic certainly has no monopoly on primary care. At least as many as are on its registered lists utilise either the services of their ISAPREs, or of such external donor-driven health centres as the *Fundación Cristo Vive* supported *Centro en Salud Familia* community health centre. There is direct, unfettered access here to the individual specialists who operate privately in their own premises rather than within the nurse and social work-triaged confines of San Joaquín.

Nevertheless, the San Joaquín polyclinic is expanding. It now has three quali-fied dentists as full-time employees, a rarity in South America and elsewhere. Its psychologists receive as many direct referrals as any of the other profession-als; also an exceptional occurrence. The roles of the nutritionist and the dispenser are underpinned by standard national requirements for minimum supply and safety, while the status of social assistants is raised with their health professional peers by a mandatory five-year pre-registration training period and reduced wage differentials. These have been negotiated by the national 21 000-member multiprofessional trade union in which community nurses have been particularly prominent. The trade union holds both the power of the short-term strike and the long-term deal. It is a crucial partner in Chile's pioneering strate-gies for the reformed polyclinic in primary care.

Its multiprofessional profile and interests have helped to ensure that no indi-vidual specialism has skewed the overall balance of interests at such primary care organisations as that of San Joaquín. Here it is a female physiotherapist who has been selected as the executive director, while one of the doctors serves as clinical lead on the Area Council overseeing the needs and provision for a 60 000 population. The aim nationally is for three general medical practitioners for every 10 000 people. But only seven of 14 medical schools provide the curriculum for a specialism that was validated only in 1993. There are just 240 GPs nationwide and the export trade in qualified medical personnel is flourish-ing, so that the Ministry of Health has had to compensate for native losses with up to a third of foreign recruits to family doctor positions in its pioneer projects.

At the main Catholic University in Santiago the Dean of Medicine has recog-nised the *realpolitik* of the situation. In 2003/04 as few as 14 of the GP vocational training places were taken up and his plans for 'super specialists' in family medicine are now subsumed within a support framework of research and development for San Joaquín and the other reformed polyclinic initiatives. It is, in his view, and the words of the national director of primary care, more impor-tant to support a 'long-term silent revolution away from the biomedical to the psychosocial' than it is to back any one generalist discipline. While attempts elsewhere to adopt a similar mixed model seem to have stalled (e.g. in Argentina),[7] a public service network of reformed polyclinics influenced and sharpened by private practice, enhanced by more qualified general medical practitioners and fundamentally multiprofessional, is seen to offer the best prospect of delivering such a revolution for Chile.

Chile	
1 Capital city:	Santiago
2 Demographic factors:	
Population size (million)[a]	16.3 (2005)
Age profile[a]	7.6% (aged < 5), 8.1% (aged 65 and over) (2005)
Ethnicity[b]	White and white-Amerindian 95%; Amerindian 3%; other 2%

3 Socioeconomic factors:
   GDP per capita (International $)[c]   11 086 (2002)
   Health expenditure per capita
   (International $)[c]   642 (2002)
   Health expenditure per GDP[c]   5.8% (2002)
   Main industry[b]   Copper; other minerals; foodstuffs;
                                        fish processing; iron and steel;
                                        wood products; transport equip-
                                        ment; cement; textiles

4 Health factors:
   Life expectancy at birth[c]   77.0 (M 74.0/F 88.0) (2003)
   Five main causes of death
   (rate per 100 000 population)[d]   Diseases of circulatory system,
                                        146.99; neoplasms, 124.35; exter-
                                        nal causes, 81.05; diseases of respi-
                                        ratory system, 55.33; diseases of
                                        digestive system, 41.17 (2001, ICD
                                        10 used, coverage rate 100.0%)

5 Organisational factors:
   Primary care model   Municipally managed with a
                                        generic multiprofessional primary
                                        care team model, small and private
                                        general practices and clinics
   Resources (health personnel)[e]   11.5 physicians/10 000 pop. (1998);
                                        6.6 nurses and midwives/10 000
                                        pop. (2003)
   Financing[j]   Local taxation; compulsory
                                        contributions for public insurance
                                        (National Health Fund: FONASA)
                                        and for private insurance
                                        (ISAPREs); income from opera-
                                        tions; out-of-pocket payments;
                                        external loans and donations
   Lead primary care practitioners   Multispecialists in family medicine

Policy priorities
A *Universal access to care through intersectoral approach (public-private, health-social)*
   New plan AUGE (2004–), a universal health insurance with compen-
   satory fund between FONASA and ISAPREs based on risk
   management; aims to increase level of primary care; guarantees access
   to 56 priority services package; promotion of universal care by GPs
   within primary care networks; shifting from super-specialist model to
   integrated family medicine

B *Equitable care through solidarity in financing*
Redistribution of local taxes for frontline services based on health plan financing via rurality, poverty and epidemiological assessments

C *Human resources*
Universities provide national training programmes for postgraduate family doctors, including problem-based learning and integrated adult education; interprofessional focus

D *Local participation*
Promoting new decision making at municipal councils which will manage primary care networks

E *Regulation*
Common standards and regulations between FONASA and ISAPREs; Areas coordinate with other agencies for accreditation at regional level; effective tools and guidelines; establishment of national accreditation system; Mutual Cooperation Agreements between Areas and municipalities for primary care development

Future prospects

This 'best prospect' for Chile appears a good prospect for others as well. Pragmatically, the reformed polyclinic model of primary care organisation is attractive. Given reasonable financial growth and a sufficient mixed economy

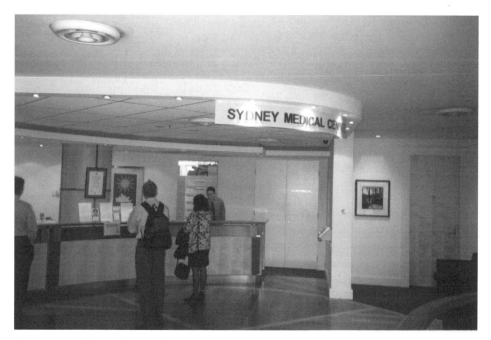

Figure 7   The Reformed Polyclinic, Sydney.

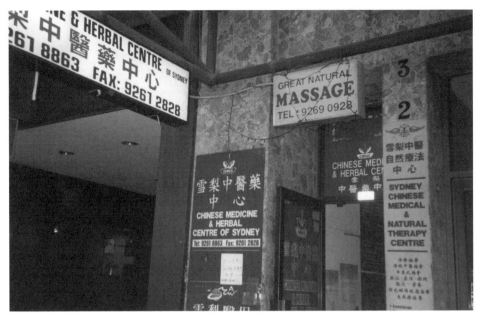

Figure 8   Chinese Medical Centre, Sydney.

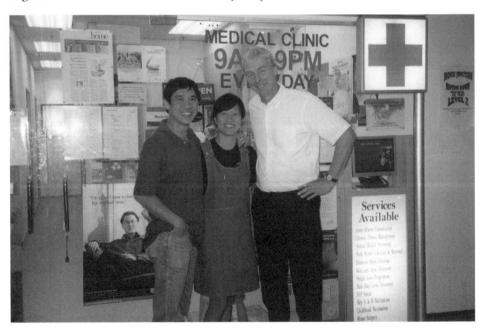

Figure 9   Singapore.

Figures 7–9 The reformed polyclinic (Australia, Australia, Singapore). The range of specialisms and service outlets is highlighted in the two photographs from the same street in central Sydney, with the mezzanine-level private medical centre on the one hand and the nearby traditional Chinese medicine practice on the other. The picture of the author and his assistants in front of a Singapore clinic indicates how the commercial drivers behind polyclinics lead to an unusual profile for such services as 'skin and acne treatment' and 'male hair loss'.

of healthcare providers with goodwill and commitment to the frontline, it offers a sustainable option both economically and socially. This view applies particularly in those places that lack the capacity for the coordination and control of commissioning that comes with the extended general practice and managed care enterprise. Moreover, many public administrations are not yet logistically ready or psychologically secure enough in their own regulatory roles to endorse either of these last two types of modern primary care organisation. The reformed polyclinic offers the challenge of achieving effective cross-boundary arrangements in terms of private and professional practice, but it is simpler and essentially a provider only-focused model.

As a result, it seems to offer a surprising number of win–wins in terms of relationships. The contribution, survival and usually development of individual professions are protected, with opportunities for growth arising from either demonstrable public demand or effective public health interventions. Between professions a plausible *modus vivendi* is achieved with an acceptable public face: certainly not interprofessional but integrated at least in the use of physical amenities. Moreover, as in Brazil, the latter may pave the way for unexpected levels of community ownership leading to further public investment and additional options for policy formulation and partnerships in a decentralised State.[8]

In Chile and Singapore, governments have sought to grasp these opportunities on behalf of whole populations and, in particular, those who previously had either poor access to primary care or bypassed its services in favour of privately purchased insurance options. Sydney reveals some of the risks that remain for both of these groups if the reformed polyclinic developments lack a coherent overall strategy and effective regulation. Essentially self-interested and individualistic in their professional portfolios, they may either slide easily into the unaccountable and fragmented secondary care outreach role we describe in Chapter 8, or more deliberately develop into a specialist managed care enterprise. At the polyclinic there remains a lack of parity in all the organisational relationships and, not least, those with patients. Primary care is at the particular provider's behest, subject to his or her practice's terms of reference and invoices. Its future should be as a staging post. It constitutes a phase of transition towards one or other of the more profound primary care organisationally ideal types we discuss in this book. It is not an end in itself.

References

1 Collins C, Aravjo J, Barbosa J (2000) Decentralising the health sector: issues in Brazil. *Health Policy.* **52**: 113–27.
2 Batterham R, Southern D, Appleby N et al. (2002) Construction of a GP integration model. *Social Science and Medicine.* **54**: 1225–41.
3 Marjoribanks T, Lewis J (2002) Reform and autonomy: perceptions of the Australian general practice community. *Social Science and Medicine.* **56**: 2229–39.
4 Hall J (1999) Incremental change in the Australian health care system . *Health Affairs.* **18**(3): 95–110.
5 Britrán R, Muñoz J, Aguad P et al. (2000) Equity in the financing of social security for health in Chile. *Health Policy.* **50**: 171–96.
6 Bertranov F (1999) Are market-oriented health insurance reforms possible in Latin America? *Health Policy.* **47**: 19–36.

7 Barrientos A, Lloyd-Sherlock P (2000) Reforming health insurance in Argentina and Chile. *Health Policy Plan.* **15**(4): 417–23.

8 Castañeda T (1997) *Health Sector Reforms in Brazil: decentralization to States and Municipalities.* Washington, DC: World Bank.

Country profile sources

Singapore, Brazil, Australia and Chile

[a] Population Division of the Department of Economic and Social Affairs of the United Nations Secretariat (2005) World Population Prospects: The 2004 Revision Population Database. http://esa.un.org/unpp/ (accessed 22/06/05).

[b] Central Intelligence Agency (2005) The World Factbook. www.cia.gov (accessed 27/06/05).

[c] World Health Organization (2005) Core Health Indicators, WHO Statistical Information System. www.who.int (accessed 23/06/05).

[d] Adapted from World Health Organization (2005) WHO mortality database. www.who.int (accessed 08/09/05).

[e] World Health Organization (2005) World Health Statistics 2005, WHO Statistical Information System. www.who.int (accessed 23/06/05).

[f] World Bank (2003) Financing health care: Singapore's innovative approach. http://rru.worldbank.org/Documents/PublicPolicyJournal/261Taylo-050803.pdf (accessed 03/09/05).

[g] Martinez J (1999) Brazil: health briefing paper. London: DFID Health Systems Resource Centre. www.dfidhealthrc.org/shared/publications/Country health/BRAZIL.PDF (accessed 05/09/05).

[h] De A Custodio F, Andrade F (2001) *The Brazilian Healthcare Sector.* Rio de Janeiro: British Consulate-General.

[i] Hilless M, Healy J (2001) *Health Care Systems in Transition, Australia.* The European Observatory on Health Care Systems. Copenhagen: EOHCS. www.euro.who.int/observatory (accessed 24/08/05).

[j] Pan American Health Organization (1999) *Profile of the Health Services System: Chile.* Program on Organization and Management of Health Systems and Services. Washington, DC: Pan American Health Organization.

Chapter 6

The district health system

Introduction

The component features of the district health system (DHS) make sense to everybody. Regular and comprehensive needs assessments; pooled resources across public and private sectors; sound public administration and interventions targeted at the poor and least privileged: who could argue with any of these? The DHS problem, however, has been that although the idea appeals to everybody, in its implementation there is not enough for anybody. And certainly not for any of those political, professional or provider units that are accustomed to taking forward health services, including primary care. The family doctor, for example, is usually relegated upstairs to a third-tier strategic oversight position. The local councillor or national minister is expected not to make decisions for his or her communities but to share leadership with non-governmental agencies whose patrons may be both remote and of very different persuasions. And the general practice and hospital are somehow both felt to be an anathema in seeking funds and posts that respond to the felt needs of those coming through their outpatient, emergency and surgery doors, because their patients' morbidity profiles do not chime with the analyses of district epidemiologists and directors of public health. Above all the DHS, paradoxically, is not viewed as locally manufactured, but a one-size-fits-all product of the WHO for which sub-Saharan Africa was the main unwitting and defenceless recipient. And look what (mostly) happened there.

As the following case exemplars demonstrate, however, it should not be written off by either developing or developed countries. Its intellectual coherence provides principles which, at the very least, are reference points for all organisational developments in primary care. In practice, as our Pallisa and Medelin research suggests, it can achieve really major and rapid improvements in health status and resource capacity. These macro-level transformations should also not disguise significant micro-developments, especially in terms of successful substitution for medical and even nursing professional roles and the revised training inputs these then require. Both South Africa and the Czech Republic are discovering this, even if the two case exemplars from these countries in this chapter suggest faltering progress.

The DHS is probably best regarded as a twentieth-century legacy. In international terms, the twin forces of regionalism and globalisation are clearly better suited, for example, to the community development agency and managed care enterprise respectively. But the DHS remains too important to too many powerful interests, and too influential in practice, however patchy its prospects, to set aside at this stage. Like the extended general practice, when policy makers and professionals think about modern primary care organisational developments and the 'multiple forces' that shape them,[1] the portable notion of a district health system with all the controls it seems to offer is still from where they start.

Pallisa

With the exception of the war-torn areas of the north, Pallisa in eastern Uganda is the poorest of the 45 districts in the country. Its rural economy is devoid of natural resources and historic investment. Its population is just under three-quarters of a million, for whom there are just four doctors working away from the 100-bed Pallisa District Hospital in local community settings. This is 10% of the total medical establishment and actually fewer than the number of doctors who have places on the 15-member management board for the DHS. They number six. Yet primary care services and their development are genuinely what is termed a Priority Programme Area for this executive, having been defined as such in the 1997 national Poverty Eradication Action Plan (PEAP) and the subsequent post-2000 seven- and three-year national and local strategies of the Kampala government's Decentralisation Secretariat for capacity building in the DHS. A series of primary healthcare conditional grants are designed to double the number of qualified healthcare personnel to two-thirds of the local workforce by 2005/06.[2]

This approach to capacity building looks to blend internal and external contributions in pursuit of synergies that may, at least partially, overcome major shortfalls in resources. Some of the negotiations for the PEAP took place in Geneva, and both the WHO Provider Directorate and World Bank were influential in achieving agreement on the targeted provision of a Minimum Health Care Package in Uganda through what the UK government termed a 'Sector-Wide Approach' (SWAp). Under the terms of this SWAp, such official outside donors as the Danish International Aid Agency have, for example, underwritten for some districts basic drugs procurement and prescribing programmes.[3] In Pallisa, annual State expenditure remains minimal, at less than $8 per capita, and less than half the total spend on healthcare, but it has at least doubled in five years.

This external expansion has been more than matched by the growth generated within the DHS from its own native resources. The key to this success story has been the pitching of five levels of primary care provision at five levels of existing social infrastructure and community organisation. Moreover, at each of these levels exists a level of legitimate and indeed even democratic authority which it has been possible to co-opt and incorporate into the overall district health system. The significance of this approach in terms of communicating effective political messages and disease prevention can scarcely be overstated during a time when both AIDS/HIV and malaria have been particularly virulent threats. Uganda's record on both has been impressive.

This is a testimony to its model of primary care organisation. Ugandan decentralisation dates back to legislation in 1959 and was solidified by the post-Amin 1987 Health Policy Review Commission, which firmly established local districts as the level for 100-bed general hospitals.[4] The congruence with community structures in terms of provision is complemented by a similar cultural fit in terms of commissioning. At the top, the fifth district level, executive committee representation is across education, agriculture, production, works, finance and community development with elected and appointed members exercising corporate responsibility for the integration of district facilities including the general hospital. The committee has a dedicated 15-strong health management team which includes, since 1996/97, one or more persons from the district panel of contributory non-governmental organisations. At the other end, Level 1, the parish, these may be the principal or only primary care providers, often as an integral part of the role of mission churches. Other personnel on the district health management team include officers responsible for health education, infection control, reproductive and environmental health, drugs procurement and prescribing, as well as five subdistrict medical representatives and the hospital superintendent. This committee has custodianship of the DHS. Its fundamental role is to ensure the most effective and equitable distribution of human resources and service outlets. To these ends it now possesses annual licensing powers in respect of NGOs and the capacity to raise local health taxes in support of its immunisation campaigns and targets for personnel recruitment. It has the authority to amend and extend the 13 objectives set out in the national Priority Programme.

Levels 2–4 are, in order: the subcounty or village(s); the county, which is the main assembly of elected councillors, again often with parallel NGO representation; and the subdistrict. Each level also fits with a grade of health centre, the status reflecting population coverage and professional profiles. Kadama Health Centre, for example, provides for 37 000 people and is open 24 hours a day. Operational leadership comes from one of Makerere University's three-year-trained community practitioner clinical officers and the staff include two midwives, a nurse and two nursing aids and assistants. There are two delivery beds: new mothers are allowed up to six hours postnatal inpatient care.

At Level 2 there are no beds and no clinical officers, but in Pallisa at Level 4 health centres such as Kubuku or Buduca there are as many as 18 beds, with a population coverage of 50 000 and a doctor-led team that includes three qualified community nurses, a health educationalist as well as midwives and auxiliaries. All levels of health centre have community management committees that include local elders, secretaries for youth and women, and designated resource 'mobilisers' and health 'educators'. Those with these titles proudly wear the coloured t-shirts bearing their nomenclatures. The county level selects its subdistrict level support which, in turn, reinforces the role of elected councillors in, for example, promoting the use of condoms or mosquito nets to combat AIDS/HIV and malaria. At Kadama, for example, one young councillor, the son of a tribal leader, vividly described how he had to explain to local village audiences of up to a hundred, the risks of HIV infection. The banana figures prominently among his visual aids for explaining the role of condoms; much to his embarrassment on the occasion when the gathering included his parents and grandparents!

The DHS has a long way to go in Uganda. It lacks local resources and planning capacity. The quality of the patient experience is unchanging, and over half of care and expenditure remains in the largely informal private sector.[5] But the DHS has achieved a political consensus, popular credibility and a real level of multiprofessional goodwill. This has allowed universities like Makerere, or Moi at Eldoret in Kenya across the border, to pioneer Community Based Education and Service (COBES) models whereby trainee doctors, nurses and pharmacists from Year 1 undertake and design community placements together as an essential part of their pre-registration training. In Uganda, the aim of the Mulaga School of Public Health in Entebbe is training centres for community practice located around the country. Each would cover 150 000 catchment areas in a hub-and-spoke model with Makerere University at Kampala. With backing from the Rockefeller Foundation and no fewer than seven Ministry of Health representatives on the Vice Chancellor's Decentralisation Committee it might even happen. The problems of poverty in Uganda should not disguise the richness of the potential. The DHS organisational model for primary care in Pallisa is a relative success.

Uganda

1 Capital city: Kampala

2 Demographic factors:
  Population size (million)[a]   28.82 (2005)
  Age profile[a]   20.7% (aged < 5), 2.5% (aged 65 and over) (2005)
  Ethnicity[b]   Baganda 17%; Ankole 8%; Basoga 8%; Iteso 8%; Bakiga 7%; Langi 6%; Rwanda 6%; Bagisu 5%; Acholi 4%; Lugbara 4%; Batoro 3%; Bunyoro 3%; Alur 2%; Bagwere 2%; Bakonjo 2%; Jopodhola 2%; Karamojong 2%; Rundi 2%; non-African (European, Asian, Arab) 1%; other 8%

3 Socioeconomic factors:
  GDP per capita (International $)[c] 1038 (2002)
  Health expenditure per capita
  (International $)[c]   77 (2002)
  Health expenditure per GDP[c] 7.4% (2002)
  Main industry[b]   Sugar; brewing; tobacco; cotton textiles; cement; steel production

4 Health factors:
  Life expectancy at birth[c]   49.0 (M 47.0/F 50.0) (2003)
  Five known main causes of death[d] Perinatal and maternal conditions, 20%; malaria, 15.4%; acute lower respiratory tract infections, 10.5%; HIV/AIDS, 9.1%; diarrhoea, 8.4% (1995)

5 Organisational factors:
    Primary care model   Five-level district health system
                                          with elected management and
                                          stratified local health centre
                                          provision
    Resources (health personnel)[e]   0.5 physicians/10 000 pop. (2002);
                                          0.9 nurses and midwives/10 000
                                          pop. (2002)
    Financing   External donors funds; central
                                          government grants; local revenue
                                          contributions; out-of-pocket
                                          payments
    Lead primary care practitioners   Community nurses

Policy priorities[f]
A *Communicable diseases*
  HIV/AIDS and malaria control programmes implemented at district
  level
B *Partnerships*
  Effective international partnerships between government and NGOs
  through the Sector-Wide Approach (SWAp)
C *Decentralisation*
  Through the health subdistricts and counties; fiscal decentralisation
  and partnership management; 'Priority Programme' block grants for
  primary healthcare with selective national performance indicators
D *Human resource development*
  Community-oriented new curricula for nursing and dentistry; central
  financial support (sponsorships) for education of health professionals
  and higher wage levels than private sector to avoid brain drain;
  promotion of volunteer community health workers and
  bicycles/motorcycles to outreach remote communities; development of
  local capacity building through community training centres
E *Restructure*
  Shifting role of national government to policy development, regulation and technical assistance

Mathbestad

As a State, post-Apartheid South Africa is starting over. Article 27 of its new
Constitution in 1996 asserted the right of universal free access to healthcare
services and the duty of the State 'to take reasonable legislative measures within
available resources'. To exercise these new responsibilities the governments of
Nelson Mandela and Tabo Mbeke have opted for the DHS model. The aim has
been renewal through policies of growth, employment and redistribution
(GEAR), in which all resources, including those of professionals, are pooled in
the interests of community regeneration. The new Constitution and Bill of

Rights were quickly reinforced by a 1997 White Paper on the 'Transformation' of the health system[6,7] and the launch of 22 nationwide reconstruction programmes. Within three years the DHS health reform initiative had produced 700 new or refurbished primary care clinics, and the principle of 'distributional justice' had, it seemed, been put into practice.[8]

The Mathbestad Clinic, an hour and a half's drive across the plains from Johannesburg, is one of these clinics. It serves the nationally prescribed standard population of 10 000 and is the main health facility for one of Moretele's four subdistricts. Its appearance is a mirror image of modern South Africa. Lots of land with a small garden-produce allotment on the site and the main clinic in a long low building with bare walls and basic consulting and waiting rooms that have seen better days. Local lads lounge by the trees and some young mothers sell assorted produce and first aid items at the entrance, plus, extraordinarily, an immaculate but little-used separate Medical Training Centre with the logo of a major international pharmaceutical company prominently displayed on its front wall. And in the surrounding area a small township with 40% unemployment, caravan-style, tin-built abodes and, incredibly, small but private clinics also scattered around, sometimes opening for business for as little as a few hours a week.

These clinics include those of some family medical practitioners. There are no doctors based at Mathbestad. The nearest recognisable general practices are 100 kilometres or more away at the universities of Pretoria and Medunsa. An academic GP does call in at the clinic most weeks and this association has led to the accreditation of Mathbestad as a training unit for trainee doctors. However, the clinic is not their show; it is unequivocally now that of the nurses. In 1996 this was not the intention, but ten years later 'the triple-trained nurse' – health promoter/clinician/therapist – has professionalised the DHS in South Africa and made it her property.

At Mathbestad there is a sister-in-charge, two primary healthcare nurse sisters and then a team of nursing assistants who ensure 24-hour staffing. They all report to the district nursing officer. A thousand miles away in the township of Lange at the newly built Bundeheuwal Community Health Centre we visited in 2003, the model is the same. This time the more recently initiated service model has been deliberately designed with protocol-driven nurse triage, prescribing and public health programmes for this densely populated part of western Cape Town. Here the metamorphosis of the district health system is clearly evident. Bundeheuwal covers three times the population of Mathbestad, and as 30 000 has become the Cape Town norm so its 'equity gauge' for efficient resource redistribution has led to regular reductions in the number of city districts from 11 to eight to four.

Such a rationalisation recognises the realities that South Africa does not have the social structures and strengths of, for example, Uganda to sustain a local community-based model of primary care organisation. Its national Health Professions Council remains conservative, secondary care and profit-oriented. Even the Medical Training Unit at Mathbestad is a product of the Rural Health Initiative run by the Academy of Family Practice in conjunction with businesses incentivised by corporate tax exemptions. The post-1996 Durban-based Progressive Primary Care Network, which campaigned vigorously for country-wide multiprofessional primary healthcare, is now almost exclusively focused on Kwazulu Natal Province, as the sponsoring funds from the Kaiser Foundation have run out. The same applies to the Rodenbosch Health Systems Trust, previously backed by the Kellogg Foundation, which also powerfully supported proposals for local clinical capacity building and shifts away from private healthcare in its challenging and much-respected Annual Health Review Reports after 1996.[9] It now fears that South African primary care will subside into a set of vertically managed public health programmes with minimal community support or development and community nursing as a vehicle for medical substitution and African middle-class aspirations. The DHS could descend, as in Tanzania, to merely 'selective healthcare' with supermarket-style packages of healthcare goods.[10]

Back in the districts of both Moretele and Lange there is evidence to back up this thesis. Together their administrative officers speak of 200 post-qualification doctors leaving the country to live and work abroad in the past year, and the medical personnel we met in the local clinics were Dutch, German, Iranian and Cuban. The City Health Director tells us his role model in the past for the organisation of primary care was either New Zealand or the UK. Now it is Bangladesh. At Mathbestad the clinical forum for local patient involvement is poorly attended and here, as elsewhere, plans for such community representative arrangements at clinic, subdistrict and district level have been abandoned. The traditional tribal chiefs in Moretele have not engaged with the process which is seen still as 'managerial' or even 'modern colonial'.

In this district, 50% of Africans go to healers first for their frontline healthcare. The national model of the district health system with its 'Integrated Development Plans' seems somehow to have missed out this reality on the one hand, while on the other in Cape Town the European population still gives the Bundeheuwal Centre a miss. They can be found down at the gentrified Alfred Docks, opposite the Business School, attending the private GP-run Greenpoint Health Centre with the facilities of the Old City Hospital on the doorstep. Worlds apart; different and distinct cultures and expectations that the DHS organisation of primary care is struggling to resolve and reconcile in South Africa.

South Africa	
1 Capital city:	Pretoria
2 Demographic factors:	
Population size (million)[a]	47.43 (2005)
Age profile[a]	11.0% (aged < 5), 4.2% (aged 65 and over) (2005)
Ethnicity[b]	Black 75.2%; white 13.6%; coloured 8.6%; Indian 2.6%

3 Socioeconomic factors:
GDP per capita (International $)[c]   7935 (2002)
Health expenditure per capita
(International $)[c]   689 (2002)
Health expenditure per GDP[c]   8.7% (2002)
Main industry[b]   Mining (platinum, gold, chromium);
                                      automobile assembly; metalworking;
                                      machinery; textile; iron and steel;
                                      chemicals; fertiliser; foodstuffs;
                                      commercial ship repair

4 Health factors:
Life expectancy at birth[c]   49.0 (M 48.0/F 50.0) (2003)
Five known main causes of death
(number of associated deaths)[g]   Tuberculosis, 56 985; influenza and
                                      pneumonia, 55 115; other forms of
                                      heart disease, 48 927; events of
                                      undetermined intent, 35 328;
                                      cerebrovascular diseases, 31 104
                                      (2001, ICD 10 used, coverage rate
                                      not defined)

5 Organisational factors:
Primary care model   Three-tier district health system
                                      model for planning and provision of
                                      services
Resources (health personnel)[e]   6.9 physicians/10 000 pop. (2001);
                                      38.8 nurses and midwives/10 000
                                      pop. (2001)
Financing   National health insurance; Medical
                                      Savings Accounts (MSAs); private
                                      health insurance funds; out-of-
                                      pocket payments
Lead primary care practitioners   Nurses

Policy priorities
A *Equality and primary care*
  Effective HIV/AIDS control and prevention programmes through new
  primary care teams; family medicine as a specialism with higher
  status; capital development of primary care clinics as part of
  Reconstruction Development Programmes (RDPs)
B *Partnerships and participation*
  New community partnerships working for HIV/AIDS through 'Multi-
  Sectoral Action Teams' including NGOs
C *Decentralisation*
  Provision of primary healthcare package through District Health
  System

D *Management and regulation*
District health information systems; provincial management to commission evaluations; promoting public-private partnership (PPP) for value-for-money and regulated mixed-economy of healthcare; new quality schemes between local clinical committees and supervisors

E *Human resource management and development*
Programmes for skills-mix nurses and community health; leaderships programmes using 'skills levy' taxes; mid-level clinical officers with medical training; registered GP training programmes with provincial accreditation and funding

Medelin

Where in South Africa there are latent tensions, in Colombia there are outright contradictions. In terms of modernising health systems, the government of Bogota can, with some justification, lay claim to global leadership with decentralisation and partnership asserted as fundamental principles in the Laws numbered 10 and 60. These paved the way for the delivery of a primary care-based Compulsory Health Plan (POS) through 1076 *municipios* as far back as 1993.[11] And yet Colombia is a country where only 0.5% of the 56 000 physicians are family doctors. When the Health Ministry was abolished in 2003 and merged with Employment in the new Ministry of Social Protection, it may have been designed as a vote of confidence in devolved government, but still less than 4% of the new central Department's Social Security General Fund was spent on community health services. This is a country where high risk is normal. Our researchers were, for example, accompanied by an armed guard throughout their fieldwork. The 'Big Bang' approach to reorganising primary care[12] has been akin at times to a battlefield and there have been casualties.

There have also been the kind of unexpected and creative developments associated uniquely with wartime. Medelin in the north of Colombia is at the forefront of these. In the absence of GPs, its elected mayors (for 50 000 populations) and medical school faculty have combined with the new Ministry, and a range of external donor agencies, including the Kellogg Foundation and World Bank, to develop a vibrant district system driven by the thematic of 'Family Health'. Its expression is essentially educative. As a policy, the notion of Family Health seeks to mobilise resources across sectors, harnessing the full range of self and statutory responsibilities for health and healthcare.

Accordingly, at the medical school it is recognised that the Colombian accelerated pace of change precludes the preparation of a new generation of family doctors with extended qualifying periods to underpin decentralisation. The Family Health aim is rather to run programmes that sensitise all physicians to local community needs and to enter into research collaborations with external and international partners, which help ensure a growing awareness of alternative and best practice. As the leading educational establishment for primary care in a country where half of the medical schools remain private hospital-based enterprises, Medelin has pioneered more-flexible entry criteria and curricula, looking to recruit cross-culturally from indigenous groups and to support the new roles of social protector and *Usuario* (new citizen). These are pivotal features across the reformed organisation of primary care. Social protectors are easily visible on their motorbikes, whether in a rural Andes region or an urban tenement. Their role is to deliver the 2001 updated POS across the community, focusing particularly on the poorer areas, refugee settlements and military casualties. The new citizens are seen as the essential counterweight to the social protectors. All three levels of health centre, from nurse outpost to community hospital with up to 50 beds, must have a *Usuarios* oversight committee and right-to-life claims of any individual have been enshrined in Colombian law since 1991, with a National Health Assembly established to receive and adjudicate on local advocacy group representations.

In Colombia, the DHS approach has led to major gains in investment, with healthcare at more than 10% of GDP in the post-millennium period. At Medelin the expansion and innovation of organisational developments in primary care point to the reasons for this growth. First there is both a public and a private version of the *Entidad Promotora de Salud* (health promotion enterprise), which receives funds through the national contributory insurance scheme. Across Colombia two-thirds of these are now private, with their own clinics and health centres. Just under half the population use them. The same proportion can access the same services through direct provision by the municipal authority on behalf of the Ministry under the terms of the POS. To support this and to augment the cover offered in Medelin as elsewhere, a network of independent health cooperatives entitled *Empresas Solidarias de Salud* have been formed at local community levels. Often in poorer areas, they can contract for either private or public healthcare services, while in some of the more affluent parts of the country, multi-municipality Collective Health Companies have also been created to offer extended and subsidised family healthcare. And, of course, in addition, there are also some, but relatively few, private direct-access and fee-for-service specialists and hospitals with, in Medelin, autonomous management and the label of State Social Enterprise. These again offer supplementary insurance options in respect of, for example, drugs provision beyond the 300 items listed in the POS nationally.

Overall, it is a dynamic organisational environment which in terms of service provision is heavily dependent on auxiliaries in, for example, nursing, oral health, laboratories and pharmacy, but is nevertheless effective in harnessing within discrete DHSs many of the available resources required to address the major threats to health that continue to include tuberculosis, dengue fever and leprosy, as well as the high prevalence of respiratory diseases and high infant mortality. In Medelin, as elsewhere, private medical practice has actually diminished with only one in 20 doctors now working outside the State system. It is an interesting contrast with the likes of Manila (*see* p.120) or even Mathbestad and Moretele (*see* p.85), and points to the potential application of the district health system model, appropriately adapted, to the organisation of primary care beyond the boundaries of the African continent.

Colombia

1 Capital city: Bogota

2 Demographic factors:
   Population size (million)[a]   45.60 (2005)
   Age profile[a]   10.4% (aged < 5), 5.1% (aged 65
                                            and over) (2005)
   Ethnicity[b]   Mestizo 58%; white 20%; Mulatto
                                            14%; black 4%; mixed black-
                                            Amerindian 3%; Amerindian 1%

3 Socioeconomic factors:
   GDP per capita (International $)[c] 6622 (2002)
   Health expenditure per capita
   (International $)[c]   536 (2002)
   Health expenditure per GDP[c]   8.1% (2002)
   Main industry[b]   Textiles; food processing; oil; cloth-
                                            ing and footwear; beverages;
                                            chemicals; cement; gold; coal;
                                            emeralds

4 Health factors:
   Life expectancy at birth[c]   72.0 (M 68.0/F 77.0) (2003)
   Five main causes of death
   (rate per 100 000 population)[h]   External causes, 137.78; diseases of
                                            circulatory system, 121.48;
                                            neoplasms, 65.03; diseases of
                                            respiratory system, 41.44;
                                            endocrine, nutritional and metabolic
                                            diseases, 22.20 (1999, ICD 10 used,
                                            coverage rate 79.3%)

5 Organisational factors:
   Primary care model   Municipally managed health centres
                                            targeting deprived areas
   Resources (health personnel)[e]   12.7 physicians/10 000 pop. (2003);
                                            6.1 nurses and midwives/10 000
                                            pop. (2003)
   Financing[i]   General taxation; national govern-
                                            ment subsidies, voluntary contribu-
                                            tions (regional, local) and compen-
                                            sation funds for subsidised insurance
                                            programme; employee contributions
                                            for contributory insurance
                                            programme; FOSYGA (Solidarity

	and Guarantee Fund) for General Health and Social Security System (SGSSS); out-of-pocket payments; mayoral levies and external loans
Lead primary care practitioners	Nursing auxiliaries plus new physicians

Policy priorities

A *Decentralisation*

Right to equitable access to healthcare services, quality of care and public health through accredited local authorities with delegated central powers

B *Partnership and participation*

Universities' strategic role from community health needs assessment to public participation in planning; multiple local partnership projects in resource generation (e.g. from community health cooperatives to subsidised Regional Health Companies); promotion of local health committees and local health advocacy groups

C *Human resources*

New (semi-) professional skills-mix; compulsory community-based training for all healthcare professions

D *Regulation*

Establishment of accreditation system for multiple payers and providers across municipalities

Prague

Just as the United Nations has been an important influence in Colombian developments, so too its ideas and association with WHO have played a part in the new post-Soviet national health structural changes of Eastern Europe and western and central Asia. During our previous research we witnessed a vast range of experimentation first hand with, for example, alternative UK- and US-style general medical practice introduced in Lithuania and Moldova[13,14] respectively, leading-edge ambulatory care in Slovenia and the use of Kyrgyzstan as a virtual laboratory for Alma Ata style public participation in the rebirth of its local health services.[15] Included in this range were versions of the district health system with the Czech Republic and Prague selected for fieldwork because of their peculiar position as the point of convergence between traditional communist values and modern Western capitalism.

This cultural mix is evident to any visitor to Prague today: the beautiful medieval squares and bridges now set alongside McDonalds and the Marriott Hotel. The Czech attempts to build DHSs that exploit its unique sense of Solidarity have also had to seek to cater for pressures arising from the advent of a market economy. Its powerful trade unions, exemplified by Prague's Medical Chambers, accordingly view health districts as much as an economic as a social unit of organisation.

Ostensibly the DHS in Prague is based on the general practice and the District Public Health Institute. This two-tier organisational model was designed simply to integrate primary medical and primary healthcare, and to incorporate over time a comprehensive home care package supported by a post-1997 social insurance scheme. In this year, all residents of Prague were required by law to enrol with a primary care doctor. Capitation payments were introduced to encourage general practice and registered local patient lists. Across the Republic 77 districts were afforded the responsibility for implementation.

By 2002/03 our interviewees from the National Public Health Association could point to some real successes. Reductions in infant mortality have been impressive, for example, and faster than the European average. But what the tourist sees when they come to Prague is not a network of community health centres and clinics. Much more apparent is the separate military hospital; the multinational companies with their own clinic facilities for their staff; the multitude of private practices; and the ambulances with the names of their host hospitals travelling round the city to recruit referrals and maintain demand. They all have their own insurance arrangements.

There are, nevertheless, general medical practitioners in Prague. Of the 80 in the country, the majority are in the capital. Most are solo and only a quarter are approved at the second 'specialist' level of qualification. In the Medical Chambers they lack status and at the University of Prague both primary care and public health as subjects are simply subsumed into the Institute of Postgraduate Studies. When we visited, in fact, neither subject had approved Masters levels programmes.

Market forces have been a significant factor in the way the organisation of Prague primary care has emerged. At an early stage, GP capitation payments were augmented by public and private fees for services. The latter include, for instance, some vaccinations and influenza inoculations. Specialist interests in the Medical Chambers have reached pacts with health insurers to retain secondary care-based treatment regimes for many chronic conditions, while some District Public Health Institutes in Prague seem to have aspired to little more than basic hygiene and sanitation standards. As a result, to achieve effective performance management for its policies the government has moved surveillance, licensing and epidemiological monitoring accountabilities upwards to 24 new regional executives, while at the local level in Prague, July 2001 legislation recognised that the private interests of health centres were such that most community health roles of prevention, rehabilitation and long-term care needed to revert back to the communes, committees of which historically sustained social structures across the city's districts.

Despite the influx of tourists the economy of Prague is still under excessive pressure. The costs of new technologies in hospitals have precluded investment in a city-wide primary care infrastructure. The laws of supply and demand have so far played into the hands of the medical profession, although the Prague Nursing School is beginning to generate a new body of community nurse practitioners. The lack of probity, as well as private interests, are real issues, and allegations of corruption and cartels are not infrequent. In Prague, the idealism that characterises the DHS as an organisation model for modern primary care is clearly tarnished with, most critically of all, the numbers of community volunteers and agencies involved in local services in decline.

Czech Republic

1 Capital city: Prague

2 Demographic factors:
   Population size (million)[a]   10.22 (2005)
   Age profile[a]   4.4% (aged < 5), 14.2% (aged 65
                                         and over) (2005)
   Ethnicity[j]   Czech 90.4%; Moravian 3.7%;
                                         Slovak 1.9%; other 4% (2001)

3 Socioeconomic factors:
   GDP per capita (International $)[k]   16 020 (2002)
   Health expenditure per capita
   (International $)[k]   1118 (2002)
   Health expenditure per GDP[k]   7.0% (2002)
   Main industry[j]   Metallurgy; machinery and equip-
                                         ment; motor vehicles; glass;
                                         armaments

4 Health factors:
   Life expectancy at birth[k]   75.0 (M 72.0/F 79.0) (2003)
   Five main causes of death
   (rate per 100 000 population)[h]   Diseases of circulatory system,
                                         560.27; neoplasms, 283.24; external
                                         causes, 114.35; diseases of
                                         respiratory system, 46.20; diseases
                                         of digestive system, 43.48 (2002,
                                         ICD 10 used, coverage rate 100%)

5 Organisational factors:
   Primary care model   Contracted GPs (with health insur-
                                         ance funds) working at municipal-
                                         ity-owned health centres with major
                                         private practice and District Public
                                         Health Institutes
   Resources (health personnel)[m]   35.2 physicians/10 000 pop. (2003);
                                         102.1 nurses and midwives/10 000
                                         pop. (2003)
   Financing[n]   Mainly employer and employee
                                         contributions for compulsory health
                                         insurance; taxation; out-of-pocket
                                         payments
   Lead primary care practitioners   GPs and public health specialists

Policy priorities
A *Public health improvement*
   District-level mixed economies of providers for local communes under
   public health districts and direction
B *Recentralisation*
   Recentralised performance management roles shifting to regions from
   districts, with local healthcare market development
C *Management and regulation*
   Strengthen the GP gatekeeper referring role to relieve overuse of
   specialist services, quality control of private sector
D *Human resource development*
   Human resource development through integrated education
   programmes including joint courses between nursing and medical
   schools

Future prospects

The prospects for the district health system are not as positive as they were even
a decade ago. Designed as a development technique, it now often stands
discredited and even disproved as such. As a social organisation its relationships
have been ideological rather than personal. Neither professions individually and

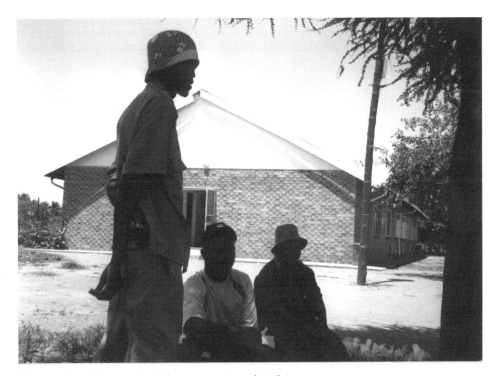

Figure 10   District health system, South Africa.

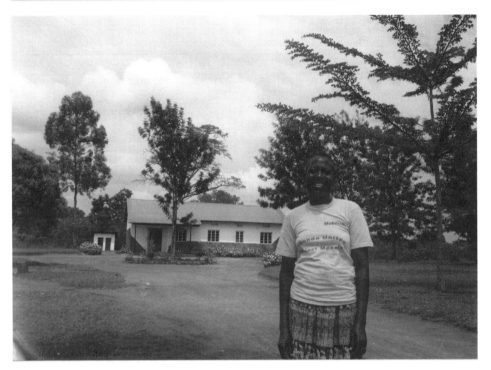

Figure 11   Pallisa, Uganda.

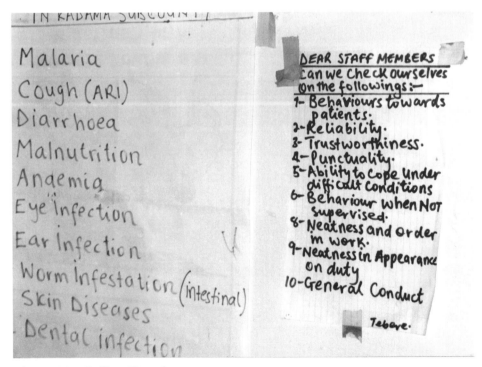

Figure 12   Pallisa, Uganda.

Figures 10–12 The district health system (South Africa, Uganda, Uganda). The two images from the Kadama Health Centre in the Uganda district of Pallisa illustrate clearly the focus on public health priorities alongside the local approach to quality standards. The local nurse featured proudly wears the t-shirt of the community's nominated 'mobiliser' for the national measles vaccination campaign. The photograph of the Mathbestad Health Centre in South Africa shows a pharmaceutical company-sponsored medical education centre incongruously located alongside the basic native facilities of the township style clinic.

collectively, nor patients and public representatives, have experienced DHS incentives as being sufficiently powerful to enlist them into this model for the organisation of primary care. Its appeal has been firmly and almost exclusively with policy makers and their partners, and the problem here is that too many of both of these groups have possessed only distinctly external relationships with both the providers and recipients of local health services. The DHS has too often merely become a research database.

Accordingly, the original DHS model, and its revised versions through the World Bank's post-1999 Comprehensive Development Framework for health investment, seem destined to be largely a framework for macro-economic evaluation.[16,17] This says it all. For while the Ugandan and Colombian experiences do point to some significant advances in public health status and education, the overall judgement even in these countries is of a cultural concept that is inherently an anti-cultural practice. As such, it is hard to know where its long-term future belongs.

References

1 Reich M (2002) Reshaping the State from above, from within, from below: implications for public health. *Social Science and Medicine*. **54**: 1669–75.

2 Njie H (2001) Poverty and ill health: the Ugandan national response. *Development*. **44**(1): 93–8.

3 Kipp W, Kamugisha J, Jacobs P et al. (2001) User fees, staff incentives and service utilisation in Kabarole District, Uganda. *WHO Bulletin*. **79**(1): 1032–7.

4 Okello D, Lubanga R, Guwatudde D et al. (1998) The challenge to restoring basic health care in Uganda. *Social Science and Medicine*. **46**(1): 13–21.

5 Burungi H, Mugisha F, Nsabagasami X et al. (2001) The policy on public-private mix in the Ugandan health sector: catching up with reality. *Health Policy Plan*. **16** (supplement 2): 80–7.

6 Peterson I (2000) Comprehensive integrated primary mental health care for South Africa. Pipedream or possibility? *Social Science and Medicine*. **51**: 321–34.

7 Johns D (2001) Health and development in South Africa: from principles to practice. *Development*. **44**(1): 122–8.

8 McIntyre D, Gibson L (2002) Putting equity in health back on to the social policy agenda: experience from South Africa. *Social Science and Medicine*. **54**: 1637–56.

9 Doherty J, McIntyre D, Bloom G et al. (1999) Health expenditure and finance: who gets what? *WHO Bulletin*. **77**(2): 156–9.

10 Saunders D, Chopra M (2001) Implementing comprehensive and decentralised health systems. *International Journal of Integrated Care*. **1**(2): 1–13.

11 Pan American Health Organization (2002) *Profile of Health Services System of Colombia.* Program on Organization and Management of Health Systems and Services. Washington, DC: PAHO.

12 Hearst N, Blas E (2001) Learning from experience: research on health sector reform in the developing world. *Health Policy Plan.* **16** (supplement 1): 1–3.

13 Meads G (1993) Nuts and Baltics. *Health Services Journal.* **103**(5334): 22–3.

14 Meads G, Meads P (2001) *Trust in Experience. Transferable learning for primary care trusts.* Oxford: Radcliffe Medical Press, pp.9–12.

15 Meads G (2003) Primary care trusts as laboratories of change. Notes from small countries. *Primary Care Report.* **5**(9): 19–21.

16 World Bank Institute (1999) *Development Outreach: putting knowledge to work for development.* Washington, DC: World Bank.

17 Tollman S, Zwi A (2000) Health systems reform and the role of field sites. *WHO Bulletin.* **78**(1): 125–34.

Country profile sources

Uganda, South Africa, Colombia and Czech Republic

[a] Population Division of the Department of Economic and Social Affairs of the United Nations Secretariat (2005) World Population Prospects: the 2004 revision population database. http://esa.un.org/unpp/ (accessed 22/07/05).

[b] Central Intelligence Agency: The World Factbook (2005). http://www.cia.gov (accessed 27/06/05)

[c] World Health Organization (2005) Core Health Indicators, WHO Statistical Information System. www.who.int (accessed 23/07/05).

[d] WHO/AFRO (2001) Uganda: burden of disease. www.afro.who.int (accessed 25/08/05).

[e] World Health Organization (2005) World Health Statistics 2005, WHO Statistical Information System. www.who.int (accessed 23/06/05).

[f] Uganda Ministry of Health (2005) Health Policy Statement 2001/2002. www.health.go.ug (accessed 5/09/05).

[g] Adapted from Statistics South Africa (2005) Mortality and Causes of Death in South Africa, 1997-2003: findings from death notification. Statistical release P0309.3. www.statssa.gov.za (accessed 30/08/05).

[h] Adapted from World Health Organization (2005) WHO Mortality Database. www.who.int (accessed 08/09/05).

[i] Pan American Health Organization (2002) *Profile of the Health Services System of Colombia.* Program on Organization and Management of Health Systems and Services. Washington, DC: Pan American Health Organization.

[j] Central Intelligence Agency (2005) The World Factbook (2005). www.cia.gov (accessed 19/08/05).

[k] World Health Organization (2005) Core Health Indicators, WHO Statistical Information System. www.who.int (accessed 25/08/05).

[m] World Health Organization (2005) World Health Statistics 2005, WHO Statistical Information System. www.who.int (accessed 25/08/05).

[n] European Observatory on Health Systems and Policies (2002) Health Care Systems in Transition HiT summary Czech Republic. www.euro.who.int/observatory (accessed 25/08/05).

Chapter 7

The community development agency

Introduction

Personally, I find the community development agency the most exciting and enticing of the six organisational models outlined in this book. Its liberal, almost left-wing link with basic human rights seems to make the notion of an 'ideal type' especially apt in this case. Yet in reality this primary care organisation is always messy. Participation is the basic ethic here and inevitably this means that while lay representations and contributions can be significantly enhanced, so too can the power afforded minorities, vested interests, corrupt cartels and even unrepresentative community factions. It is no surprise to discover an abundant research pointing to government frustrations with community development agencies.[1] Elsewhere, in settings as far apart as the Netherlands and Korea, this has led to a central reassertion of resource management and regulatory controls in pursuit of restored public trust.[2,3]

But when the community development agency works, it is a delight to witness. One of my researchers went to Peru for a week, visited Chiclayo, and then went back for four months to be among the CLAS (*Comunidades Locales de Administración de Salud*). Another enjoyed a similar experience in the 'healthy cantons' of Costa Rica. Perhaps this attraction is because in so many Western and developed countries it is participation that is the Achilles heel. In a parallel study to the present one, we found that 'local engagement' and 'public involvement' were regarded by the leaders of NHS primary care trusts as not only their weakest characteristic, but also the area where they would benefit most from exchanges with colleagues overseas.[4] It remains curious how little influence South America still has beyond its shores, but in the twenty-first century the case exemplars that follow in San José, Chiclayo, Puebla and La Paz seem bound to have their imitators elsewhere.

There are sound practical as well as idealistic reasons for thinking that this will be the case. The community development agency can go a long way towards ensuring that healthcare expenditure and priorities become less of a political burden for hard-pressed national governments. By defining themselves not in terms of healthcare but as essentially 'social organisations' they, with one leap, overcome the barriers that other models put up in terms of access to both informal and other sector investments. The much stronger contribution from women alone is a massive gain. Without hesitation then: the community development agency must be a model that merits more careful attention, rigorous scrutiny and research. It is inspirational.

Chiclayo

At our briefings with two of the most experienced directors of the World Health Organization we were advised that Peru and Bolivia set the pace for public participation in healthcare around the world. Local exemplars from these two countries top and tail this chapter. At the Geneva meetings the different styles of the two countries were emphasised and our case studies illustrate their alternative approaches, with the Lima government facilitating what it terms 'a systemic development', while its La Paz counterpart relies more on precise legislative programmes to structure local engagement. What both countries share is a fundamental commitment to health as an integral part of civil society. As the lead policy maker for primary care in Peru told us: 'We see health as a "citizen" not a "profession" issue. Mature government and social participation go together'.

Chiclayo in northwest Peru is an unlikely location as a laboratory for the changes in primary organisation that such a policy position requires. Dusty, dirt track streets, downtrodden tenements and domestic violence referrals are the context for its Urugauna Health Centre. Yet the photographs we took tell a different story (*see* p.116). The infectious vitality and enthusiasm of the 50 or so local volunteer community health agents comes across. Wearing blue t-shirts and clearly drawn from across the generations of the 12 000 neighbourhood population, they dominate the picture. The medical director and the other GP are swamped and the six midwives and nurses perch on the margins of the group photograph. Perhaps significantly it is the armed and smartly uniformed security guard who is pressed by the local health agents to take centre stage for the camera. Handsome he may be, but it is also through him that the precious gains achieved by this MaxSalud clinic in terms of drugs and disease prevention programmes receive the necessary protection in what can still be a relatively lawless land. The community development agency model for primary care at the time of our research in 2003 existed in only 15 of the country's departments, and at the time of our visit, guerrilla activities had resumed in the neighbouring region to Chiclayo. As a leading member of ForoSalud, the national assembly organisation for the 760-plus *Comunidades Locales de Administración de Salud* (CLAS health communities) suggested: 'We are not going to have good government in health in Peru unless there is social control.' The behaviour of the Urugauna community health agents implicitly acknowledged this.

They are among the 50-plus additional primary care workers that MaxSalud, a not-for-profit foundation, has recruited since its inception in 1997 to work alongside its GPs at its three centres in Chiclayo. They serve a 50 000 population and, with some local variations, adopt the classic CLAS management model of seven-person local committees, including a clinical director as lead executive and six lay members: three locally elected and three locally appointed from constituent community organisations with approval from the Ministry of Health (MINSA). This model now applies to over 2100 health centres countrywide and its growth, as a natural systemic development, led to the November 2002 Decentralisation Laws which formalised MINSA approval of what is termed a new 'social managerialism' for its post-2000 Shared Administration Programme[5] in Peru. The Ministry is itself directly responsible for health service provision for three out of four people in Peru – the rest, as employees, being covered through a 9% payroll tax by the Social Security Institute (EsSalud) – and its 1812 districts are now geographically the organisational unit for primary care.

At Chiclayo the CLAS model is writ large. MaxSalud receives the backing of USAID and the American academic oversight of Baltimore-based Johns Hopkins University. Alongside other 'Future Generations' projects it is a seedbed for developments elsewhere.[6] Until beyond 2007/08 it does not have to be completely self-funding, so it can pilot different initiatives to explore the viability of converting community participation into constructive and enduring community development. So far the different local and international evaluations of the CLAS model have been encouraging both in terms of raised resource levels and improved public health status.[7,8] Patient satisfaction rates are demonstrably sound and at Chiclayo, MaxSalud has pioneered, for example, the low-cost sale of basic domestic drugs supplies, prepayment maternity packages, nominal consultation fees and cooperative local health insurance schemes. Its economic policies, which include CLAS control of pharmaceuticals procurement and local pricing, are derived from mapping the social capital of neighbourhoods and a detailed community health diagnosis, which utilises the soft intelligence of the centre agents as well as hard epidemiological data. The basic principles are that of capacity building and shared responsibility and ownership: *'Cógestion de los Servicios de Salud'*; leading to what is called two-dimensional *'Calidad'*. As a result, each consultation of around 20 minutes, the clinic director asserts, should balance the pursuit of good clinical outcomes with personal respect and dignity. MaxSalud itself, at the level of its board, places 'Community participation' alongside 'Health promotion' and 'Curative care' as the headings for its presidential executive functions. In a country where culturally *'machismo'* and *'clientelismo'* have been prevalent features, as a result of powerful military and often corrupt political elites, this amounts to a novel and liberal exercise of authority.

The Chiclayo developments were among the 1200 new clinics that created a national infrastructure for primary care in Peru in the years after a national Fund for Development and Social Cooperation was created (1991–97). Across Peru this embraced local 'service circles', elders and, in particular, such women's health groupings as the *Movimiento Manuela Ramos*; plus in some areas members of the Roman Catholic and evangelical church communities. All of these constituencies are now significantly represented in the CLAS and MINSA local management arrangements, and together Ministry officials describe their impact in reducing 'doctor autonomy and resistance'. The Ministry itself has made its decentralisation a practical reality through district-level accountability for six new national health programmes, some of which have required new district social insurance payments across the country (e.g. for school and maternal health). A consultant (both managerial and medical) to MINSA described to us the importance of the government itself working together through its various parts as a role model for *Seguro Integral de Salud*. It is a laudable proposition with the head of Health Partnership Reforms in Lima outlining no fewer than 50 new proposals, including more joint educational curricula, during our time with her.

Ultimately, as in Bolivia, Peru does not believe in a separate organisation for primary care. This would risk professional capture and regulation. Its community development agencies are wider in their remit as a societal dynamic. It would be dangerous to divide them into constituent parts and the role of the *Defensoría del Pueblo* who oversees providers nationally is not to protect health services *per se* but to preserve human rights. From this perspective primary healthcare is fundamental.

Peru

1 Capital city: Lima

2 Demographic factors:
   Population size (million)[a]   27.97 (2005)
   Age profile[a]   10.7% (aged < 5), 5.3% (aged 65 and over) (2005)
   Ethnicity[b]   Amerindian 45%; mestizo (mixed Amerindian and white) 37%; white 15%; black, Japanese, Chinese and other 3%

3 Socioeconomic factors:
   GDP per capita (International $)[c]   5101 (2002)
   Health expenditure per capita
   (International $)[c]   226 (2002)
   Health expenditure per GDP[c]   4.4% (2002)
   Main industry[b]   Mining and refining of minerals and metals; petroleum extraction and refining; natural gas; fishing and fish processing; textiles; clothing; food processing

4 Health factors:
   Life expectancy at birth[c]   70.0 (M 68.0/F 73.0) (2003)
   Five main causes of death
   (rate per 100 000 population)[d]   Diseases of circulatory system, 113.4; neoplasmas, 112.2; acute respiratory infections, 68.2; external causes, 63.5; diseases of urinal system, 25.0 (2000, ICD 10 used, coverage rate 47.9% considered in calculation)

5 Organisational factors:
   Primary care model   Shared Administration Programme (Ministry of Health and community representatives); community health agents outreach from local committees and clinics

---

Resources (health personnel)[e]	11.7 physicians/10 000 pop. (2000); 8.0 nurses and midwives/10 000 pop. (2000)
Financing	Taxation; out-of-pocket payments; Peruvian Social Security Institute (EsSalud) (9% premium of salary); premiums paid by the non-poor for the Comprehensive Health Insurance (SIS); private insurance funds; external loans and donations
Lead primary care practitioners	Community health workers

Policy priorities

A *Universality, equitable and comprehensive access to healthcare*
Establishing the nationwide Comprehensive Health Insurance (SIS: *Seguro Integral de Salud*) scheme to provide free care for the extreme poor (24.4% of total population); extending eligibility of EsSalud towards informal sectors; increasing distribution of health professionals to rural and poor areas

B *Decentralisation and participation*
Implementing nationally coordinated and decentralised health system (SNCDS) (2002–) in which municipalities responsible for management of primary care and regional governments for hospitals with central guidance; establishing provincial and regional health councils; promoting social participation through representatives of grassroots organisations in local health councils

C *Partnerships*
Promoting coordination between the Ministry of Health and EsSalud at local level; promoting coordination between the Ministry of Health and the Ministry of Education to establish municipal teams in health promotion

D *Human resources*
Introducing comprehensive curricula including General Integrated Medicine at medical schools (2003–)

San José

Costa Rica is so achingly beautiful and such a 'slow jazz' culture that it comes almost as a shock that it should also be at the cutting edge of primary care organisational development around the world. A tourist's paradise, it is no surprise that its national university, located at the twin campus sites of Turialba and the capital city San José, should have the widest range of academic partners that we encountered. There are exchange links with McGill in Montreal, Rochester in New York, Buenos Aires in Argentina, Mozambique and of course Madrid and several other Spanish institutions to name just a few. Any external tender is rapidly oversubscribed and both WHO and World Bank officials are said to look to this country for their final pre-retirement placements. With this rich diversity of international intelligence and an exceptionally high level of Internet-based environmental scanning, Costa Rica has opted for the community development agency model for its primary healthcare.

And it has been unequivocally successful with a WHO millennium rating in the top 30 countries for its national health system. It has not only doubled its public expenditure on primary care to a little under 25% over ten years in 2003/04, but also increased overall annual health expenditure in the same period to 10% of GDP or $250 per capita. This achievement places Costa Rica at the forefront of Central America. Not surprisingly, it hosts the meetings of health ministerial representatives and chief officers for the six surrounding countries of this region.

Its organisational framework for primary care development is a series of tripartite agreements. The first of these relates to funding. Since 1993/94 the National Health Insurance scheme administered by the *Caja Costaricense de Seguro Social* (CCSS) has derived its income from different and variable combinations of State, employer and employee contributions, depending on the status of the last two. The government contribution is fixed and constant for all, guaranteeing universal coverage.

The second tripartite agreement relates to decision making. The CCSS actively commissions public health and healthcare for its 4.3 million population. But its proposed service contracts must attract 80% community support through the appropriate canton-level elected health *junta* and the Ministry of Health. There are 1200 of the former nationwide. The latter is responsible for health promotion and strategy.

The third three-party arrangement is in the services model of primary care itself. The *ebais* or clinic level team for 3–10 000 people must comply with national standards for care personnel, must include community members in basic provider functions and must partner an appropriate educational and administrative agency for the purposes of ongoing evaluation and development. Each *ebais* is designed to be a learning organisation with, for example, daily telemedicine link-ups with the central University Hospital in San José for training and consultation purposes. The mission of the university itself is 'To bring light and inspiration to society'. Need we say more!

Such idealism flourishes alongside a Modernisation Directorate at the Ministry which, despite some scandals, has been decidedly hard-headed in its reform programmes. The four 'pillars' for action have been:

- a weighted allocation formula to achieve national resource equity based on diagnostic related groups
- progressive targets for private capital investment in frontline public healthcare (16% over five years)
- *Pentel*-driven integrated information management systems
- effective modern public service and public health management programmes.

The last of these in San José now has 25 new graduates per annum. The comprehensive reform strategy in Costa Rica has been designed deliberately to overcome medical resistance[9] and to combat conservative forces through the application of global doctrines for community empowerment.[10]

The evidence of this modernisation abounds alongside the tripartite partnerships for primary care outlined above. At the three *ebais* we visited in Chirripo, Guadaloupe and southern San José itself, it is the national university, with its statutory duty of social action and development, which has acquired the line management of canton healthcare on three-year renewable contracts. Its *ebais* are local services, public health data sources and training units – all subject to the oversight of the local health *junta* in which senior citizens are often key members. In the remote Aboriginal territory of Chirripo, the *ebais* teams operate on peripatetic six-weekly cycles in the mountains. Even here they are always led by a fully qualified general medical practitioner and community nurse. They have their own medical records officer and pharmacy assistant and three locally trained native health technicians. With three months' initial preparation these men and women maintain the individual household health assessments, visiting on a regular cycle, administering inoculations and ensuring compliance through their knowledge of local dialects, remedies and *mores*. Some of these technicians have now been recruited and selected to join the national university's nursing and medical courses, and at the Curridabat *ebais* the director described to us further progress in community development through the incorporation of a social assistant into the primary care team and a sociologist and a microbiologist into its Action Research reference group.

There are 800-plus standard model *ebais* in 98 health areas across Costa Rica. As clusters, they receive managerial support and public health direction from the CCSS. In urban areas the *ebais* unit of coverage increases to populations of 10 000-plus, and for these Grecia has led the way as a town in winning national Healthy Canton competitions. The grassroots character of some of the applications for prizes is self-evident in their slogans: 'Care For Your Block', 'Thinking of Us: The Forum for Future Grandparents' and 'Participation as a Right'. Each canton is scored on a national league table against Costa Rica-wide performance indicators. Those managed by the university and its associates in San Diego, Montes de Oca and the areas described above have done especially well. The philosophy of primary care as a natural journey for service and education together seems to work in San José just as well as these values adopted in Eldoret (*see* p.5) or Tampere (*see* p.26).

The key to the effectiveness of the Costa Rican community development agencies is in their management and the buy-in from medical professionals. There are 1600 doctors in Costa Rica with formal management qualifications. They do not leave the country or their clinics. 'Ethical social action' is a principle and a practice. It is a country we have visited four times so far, each time with new learning for primary care development. We hope to do so again.

Costa Rica

1 Capital city: San José

2 Demographic factors:
  Population size (million)[a]   4.33 (2005)
  Age profile[a]   9.1% (aged < 5), 5.8% (aged 65 and
                                     over) (2005)
  Ethnicity[b]   White (including mestizo) 94%;
                                     black 3%; Amerindian 1%; Chinese
                                     1%; other 1%

3 Socioeconomic factors:
  GDP per capita (International $)[c] 7966 (2002)
  Health expenditure per capita
  (International $)[c]   743 (2002)
  Health expenditure per GDP[c]   9.3% (2002)
  Main industry[b]   Microprocessors; tourism; food
                                       processing; textiles and clothing;
                                       construction materials; fertilisers;
                                       plastic products

4 Health factors:
  Life expectancy at birth[c]   77.0 (M 75.0/F 80.0) (2003)
  Five main causes of death
  (rate per 100 000 population)[f]   Diseases of circulatory system,
                                       110.32; neoplasms, 78.47; external
                                       causes, 75.98; diseases of respiratory
                                       system, 31.38; diseases of digestive
                                       system, 26.33 (2002, ICD 10 used,
                                       coverage rate 79.3%)

5 Organisational factors:
  Primary care model   Standard nationwide integrated
                                       basic health team 'ebais' (*Equipos
                                       Basicos de Atención Integral de la Salud*)
                                       models (based on a GP, nursing
                                       assistant and local health techni-
                                       cians); nationwide 1200 elected
                                       health boards (*Juntas de Salud*) have
                                       legal rights of approval on health
                                       priorities for contract funds between
                                       cantons and CCSS (Costa Rica Social
                                       Security Agency, *Caja Costarricense de
                                       Seguro Social*)
  Resources (health personnel)[e]   16.0 physicians/10 000 pop. (2000);
                                       3.2 nurses and midwives/10 000
                                       pop. (2000)

| Financing[g] | Compulsory or voluntary contributions from the State, employers and employees for Costa Rican Social Security Fund (CCSS); voluntary health insurance |
| Lead primary care practitioners | GPs and local health technicians |

Policy priorities

A *Universal coverage, integrated care and redesigned primary healthcare model*
   Promoting universal coverage through *ebais*; promoting primary care-led health priorities and extended multiprofessional teams including dispensers and teachers

B *Partnerships and participation*
   Facilitating incentive mechanisms for primary care services through franchising *ebais* clinics; university local cooperatives manage some cantons' health services based on management agreements

C *Human resources*
   Educational programmes on local health management for all community health professionals and career ladders for local professional development

D *Health technologies*
   Promoting nationwide telemedicine training and use of research-based healthcare to target poorest indigenous populations

Libertador

Modern, red brick-built but shaped like the turret of a medieval castle, the *Consultorio Popular* sited in barren wasteland on the urban outskirts of Caracas resembles nothing so much as a small isolation unit in a high-security prison. As hard to break into when locked as it would be to break out of, this two-and-a-half spartan-roomed primary care clinic is the product of its circumstances. Over a weekend in the Venezuelan capital city, the number of offences that elsewhere might merit manslaughter charges as a minimum, can total a gross. Security is the first and foremost consideration if the post-1999 Presidential vision for genuinely universal primary care is to be achieved. The *Libertador Consultorio* has its physical equivalents right across the country. They are the symbol of a new democratic socialism.

Whereas in Costa Rica and Peru the aims are cultural compliance and conservation, in the *Municipio* of Libertador and the majority of poorer parts of Venezuela the political purpose is actually that of cultural construction. Prior to 2000, public service delivery had been 'brought to its knees'.[11] Integrated medicine has been adopted as a foundation stone of this construction. Since May 2003 the presidency-driven national *Barrio Adentro* movement has pushed forward relentlessly access to primary care, building on Article 122 of the new Constitution, which recognise the rights and practices of indigenous peoples. In the newly defined three-tier health system, Level 1 guarantees basic healthcare to all, through the minimum of a six-month-trained medical auxiliary, with access to prescriptions for all of the major morbidities, including diarrhoea, tuberculosis, malaria and, above all, respiratory diseases. Bypassing the resistance of the medical professions, the new frontline workers are developed in the government's own training centres, while 2500 applicants are now studying for the new five-year community medicine qualification. One new university in Caracas, the Bolivarian, has become in effect a government vehicle for its philosophy of 'extension', with a principal responsibility for training local trainers in the new model of primary care. Its counterpart out in the country is the *Francisco de Miranda* University in Falcon State. Both adhere closely to central health policy. There are very few independent research institutes and such nongovernmental organisations as the *Centro de Salud Sexual y Reproductiva* (PLAFAM) are virtually excluded from *Barrio Adentro*, being in this case dependent on Colombian backing for its urgent family planning work. It is located, significantly, in a middle-class area of Caracas.

Statism flourishes. Even moderate medical professionals are reluctant to discuss the change process, and yet this change process is one that compels community development. The management of the *Consultorio* we visited in Libertador is by a social council or health forum, representing 240 families and households or about 1000 local inhabitants. The council normally meets every eight days. Next to the *Consultorios* it runs its own *Mercal (Cooperativa)* store with basic food and amenities, including the government-prescribed drugs and first-aid supplies. In the *municipio* as a whole live 2.4 million people. There are no fewer than 1200 committees operating in parallel to our *Consultorio* health forum, each reporting regularly to regional citizenship assemblies on their response to both *Barrio Adentro* and the equivalent presidential '*Misiones*' (e.g. '*Robinson*' and '*Sucre*' in education) for community development.

Incentivised by capital grants, tax exemptions and compulsory post-qualifying placements of public service professionals in poorer areas, there are now 55 000 cooperatives approved and loosely monitored by a youthful national *Superintendente* in Venezuela. Their constituent members number from five to 15 000. Each has its own management structures as a local social organisation, permitting, for example, the incorporation nationally of the *Fe y Alegria* (Faith and Joy) and other influential grassroots Roman Catholic and religious groupings. Some of these are long established but now, as in the mountainside shanty town of Nueva Tacaguna, 10 kilometres from central Caracas, we found that they appear to be willing to surrender their historic functions to become one of the government's 587 designated new Level 2 diagnostic and treatment centres. Here there will be six 24-hour beds, a resident doctor and nurses, and ten on-call specialisms – from cardiology and gynaecology to orthodontics and psychology. There will also, of course, be a new social council, this time of 30 members. Back in 2000, notwithstanding Venezuela's tradition of 'coffee cooperatives' there were fewer than 100 such forums. The growth of the community development agency has undoubtedly been imposed, but for large parts of the country this populist presidential measure has also clearly struck a chord and the expansion is unequivocally explosive.

The same epithet might also be applied in prospect to the tactical but highly charged recruitment of overseas health professionals as change agents for *Barrio Adentro*. There were, according to the Ministry, 14 345 Cuban doctors practising in Venezuela in the early months of 2005. The doctor we interviewed at the *Libertador Consultorio* was Cuban. So was the sessional traumatologist who attended during our session. Moreover, the doctor lived in the bedsit upstairs. He expected to stay for two years. His 'Day of the Week' schedule for different primary care activities, which included individual chronic disease management clinics and domiciliary visits, seemed to have helped ease the way to a degree of local acceptance. But unlike in the San José *ebais* or the Chiclayo CLAS, there were no local community health worker recruits; just a trainee medical student and a single volunteer. The three national heads of primary care development we interviewed at the Ministry expected similarly that there would be few local takers from the Venezuelan health professions for the new Level 2 centres. At Nueva Tacaguna the Cadia Cooperative had appointed a Colombian to lead the transition of its 'House of Health' to diagnostic and treatment centre status. She is a woman. So too were the three national primary care strategists and 807 of those responsible for chairing the social councils. The Cuban association has had clear benefits in its introduction of community-based general practice and is part of a wider political agenda involving oil and aid. In short-circuiting orthodox models of community development, however, its enduring effectiveness as a method of policy implementation remains in question. And it is unlikely that academics from within Venezuela will be in a position to give the independent answers this question requires.

Venezuela

1 Capital city:	Caracas
2 Demographic factors:	
Population size (million)[a]	26.75 (2005)
Age profile[a]	10.7% (aged < 5), 5.1% (aged 65 and over) (2005)
Ethnicity[b]	Spanish; Italian; Portuguese; Arab; German; African; and indigenous peoples
3 Socioeconomic factors:	
GDP per capita (International $)[c]	5587 (2002)
Health expenditure per capita (International $)[c]	272 (2002)
Health expenditure per GDP[c]	4.9% (2002)
Main industry[b]	Petroleum; iron ore mining; construction materials; food processing; textiles; steel; aluminium; motor vehicle assembly

4 Health factors:
   Life expectancy at birth[c]   74.0 (M 71.0/F 77.0) (2003)
   Five main causes of death
   (rate per 100 000 population)[f]   Diseases of circulatory system,
                                        131.97; external causes, 115.75;
                                        neoplasms, 66.77; endocrine, nutri-
                                        tional and metabolic diseases, 30.06;
                                        infectious and parasitic diseases,
                                        24.60; (2000, ICD 10 used, coverage
                                        rate 97.2%)

5 Organisational factors:
   Primary care model   New preventive medicine model
                                        with *Consultorios Populares* (simple
                                        infrastructure) and Cuban doctors
                                        (14 345 in 2005) in marginal areas
   Resources (health personnel)[e]   20.0 physicians/10 000 pop. (2001);
                                        7.9 nurses and midwives/10 000
                                        pop. (1999)
   Financing[h]   Taxation (national, regional, local);
                                        earmarked revenues for health
                                        (regional and local); funds from
                                        Venezuelan Social Security Institute
                                        (IVSS), national petroleum company
                                        (PDVSA) and other insurance
                                        schemes; Public Health Comptroller;
                                        out-of-pocket for private services;
                                        external loans
   Lead primary care practitioners   Integrated Social Medicine practi-
                                        tioners and Simplified Medical Auxil-
                                        iaries (SMAs) in jungle areas

Policy priorities
A *Universal coverage, equitable access to healthcare and a new model of compre-*
   hensive care
   'Mision Barrio Adentro' (2004–) uses Cuban doctors and medicines by
   international agreement to provide integrated primary healthcare and
   strengthen infrastructure in marginal areas
B *Pro-poor and rights-based approaches (new Comprehensive Health Law 2001)*
   to health and social development
   Programmes of *Misiones* for the excluded population (e.g. *'Mision Barrio*
   Adentro' for health, *'Mision Sucre'* for higher degree education, *'Mision*
   Robinson' for reducing illiteracy, *'Mision Rivas'* for high school studies)
C *Health promotion and prevention*
   Vaccination, sexual education related to HIV/AIDS, and water supply

> D *Social participation, democratisation of capital and social control*
>   Indigenous Community Health Workers given six-month training as
>   Simplified Medical Auxiliaries (SMAs), peripatetic teams in Amazonas
>   region; promoting shared responsibility between the State and citizens
>   and sustainability through the promotion of cooperatives and health
>   forums
> E *Human resources*
>   Public universities including Bolivarian University promote preventive
>   medicine; General Integrated Medicine (or Integrated Social Medicine)
>   course for postgraduates to replace Cuban doctors as community
>   doctors in future
> F *Decentralisation*
>   Transferring the management roles to local level through municipali-
>   sation, with participative social councils

La Paz

Diversity. Diversity. Diversity. Diversity of cultures; diversity of providers, even
diversity of policy makers. In its organisation of primary care services the post-
dictatorship Bolivia has been quite exceptional in its single-minded
determination since 1982 to sustain not just the processes of community
involvement in decision making about health, but also the outcomes, however
varied, unexpected and uncomfortable they may be at times. In other countries
equity is a core principle applied to resources (e.g. Chile), services (e.g. France)
and health status (e.g. Scotland). In Bolivia it is unequivocally attached to
participation. At all levels, from individual patient care to that of the 2002
National Insurance Child and Maternal Health Programmes (SUMI), there must
be direct community involvement with rights of review, scrutiny and, ultimately, veto.

The legislative cornerstone of the Bolivian approach remains the 1995
Administrative Decentralisation Act and subsequent 1996 Supreme Decree No
24.303. These revived the intent of the original 1978 National Health Code to
'preserve, improve and restore the health of the population' but, for the first
time, placed the principal management responsibility with the 314 municipalities of its 11 regional departments or prefectures. A 20% transfer of central
government funds followed and these were soon tasked with the delivery, from
1998, of basic health insurance programmes nationwide in support of the
Ministry of Health and Sport's (SEDES) five-year 'To Live Better' strategy.[12] At
the millennium a formal National Dialogue for Health was launched, with local
health boards (DILOS) acting as the focal point for all informal processes of
exchange and formal processes of communication between SEDES, municipalities through their elected mayoral offices, and direct community members and
representatives.

At the Ancoraimes Health Centre on the outskirts of the La Paz *Prefectura* on
the banks of Lake Titikaka at 13 000 feet it was the DILOS – a three-person
agency – that appeared in 2005 to have decided to get rid of the local manage-

ment. Acting on behalf of and through a complex network of longstanding neighbourhood committees, women's groups and seniors' gatherings, and with the acquiescence at least of the majority of home-grown healthcare practitioners at the health centre itself, the local health board decided not to renew the contract of the previously much respected and Methodist-based Council for the Rural Andes. The health centre would revert to direct municipal management. Too much money laundering was suspected and the loss of public confidence in the centre was evident when we visited. It was mid-morning. Not a single patient was present for any of the 17 staff to attend to. The latter were dependent on the two market days per week for direct referrals. Neither reduced fee charges nor increased domiciliary visits (at two to three times per month per household) had made much difference in an area where there remains a deep-rooted suspicion of building-based healthcare, and half the population prefers to go direct to alternative practitioners. A change of management was required. It was community power rooted in its participative processes that effected the change. Remarkably, the last legacy of the Methodist Church was the construction on the site in 2004, by some of its American 'gap year' volunteers, of smart new premises for traditional medicine. These now stand empty. Traditional healers practise not in health centres but in homesteads. There could scarcely have been a clearer signal of how much the Rural Andes Council executive had lost touch. In its place the local Roman Catholic community now provides a cleaner, a security guard and a driver for the health centre.

At Ancoraimes the professional profile is relatively conventional (by Western norms): a medical 'hospital' director overseeing two general physicians, nine nurses and *'Sectores'* nursing auxiliaries, a pharmacist, dentist and three administrators in four hierarchic groupings – but the organisational relationships are not. The centre is a home to staff as well as a clinical setting. Its two twin-bedded wards are furnished like local living rooms. The Charter statements on the waiting room walls assert not the rights of patients but of the professionals to be treated with dignity and respect. It is they who feel the need to assert that 'pay and prestige' should be forthcoming. There is no such requirement for the public. The community holds the whip hand. It does things its way.

'Autonomy' is the third fundamental principle of primary care in Bolivia, alongside diversity and community participation. Expressed collectively they come together, for example, in extremely independent universities – many private – and intellectual disciplines. In Bolivia a doctor is a doctor and nothing else. Similarly with nurses and other healthcare therapists. Their professions are unequivocally self-interested member trade unions. The medical schools do not do management or policy. Primary care commissioning means nothing. Yet through the respect for diversity and community participation, autonomous health professionals in La Paz have put together world-class primary care organisations without, as in Peru or Colombia, the need to create separate units of health management. One hundred and thirty kilometres away from Ancoraimes in slum settlement-ridden El Alto, for example, is the superb CIES (*Centro de Investigeción y Educación en Salud*) Clinic with its remarkable daily health education drop-in facilities for local youth and parents. Here the overseeing community representative 'stakeholder assembly' is larger at nine members, as opposed to the three at Ancoraimes. But there are nine smaller centres and outposts in the El Alto 'hub-and-spoke' model to monitor in contrast to just three for 15 000 people in the rural counterpart.

Diversity leads to delineation and distinction in primary care functions. Not only are there very clearly marked out physical and clinical territories in the health centres of La Paz for *inter alia* paediatrics, urology, general medicine, ultrasound, *consejeria* (counselling for health education) and gynaecology, there are also primary care centres that specialise in each of these. Sexual health and maternity health are two of the most popular. The 42 cooperative credit union-based health centres of *Pro-Mujer* operating out of La Paz are the classic example. Like CIESs, *Pro-Mujer* is financed significantly by donor agencies in the US. Both, of course, are non-governmental organisations.

The range and growth of NGOs in Bolivian primary care are the inevitable consequence of Bolivian values. They always seek to respond to specific community needs. Sometimes they are community creations, although in La Paz most are donor dependent. As such they have separate governance. Diversity, participation and equity combine to discriminate as positively in favour of NGOs as they do in support of traditional medicine. In many parts of both rural and urban Bolivia it is the latter that is incorporating Western technologies, not *vice versa*. At the Ancoraimes Health Centre, for example, 80% of the State-salaried nursing staff employed traditional herbal and plant remedies in their treatments and half the national population still prefer a local healer as their first port of call.

The community development agency model of Bolivia is rich in its potential for transferable learning. The emphasis on 'partnerships for development' (SOCIOS) rather than simply 'for health', suggests a more profound philosophy than is encountered in most of Latin America, let alone in the extended general practices of the UK. The emphasis reflects the enduring nature of its public involvement laws and multi-ethnic culture as well, of course, as its low economic status. This has permitted such external donors as the World Bank and UNICEF to use the emerging democratic Bolivia as a laboratory for organisational experimentation in terms of new public health-oriented primary care models. Nevertheless, particularly in their range, their inclusion of traditional methods and their fully comprehensive range of relationships, the primary care organisations of La Paz are illustrations of what is possible in a 'modernising' country.

The caveat, of course, comes with the politics. La Paz is a city of beating drums, firecrackers and many marches. It is often not clear or certain that the central government is in charge. Over the past decade the Health Ministry has frequently had to play 'catch-up' with the projects sponsored through the main council for non-governmental agencies (PROCOSI), whether it liked it or not. Participation, diversity and autonomy strengthen horizontal and diagonal but not vertical relationships. National governments normally need the latter.

Bolivia

1 Capital city: Sucre (official) and La Paz (administrative)

2 Demographic factors:
Population size (million)[a]   9.18 (2005)
Age profile[a]   13.5% (aged < 5), 4.5% (aged 65 and over) (2005)
Ethnicity[b]   Quechua 30%; mestizo (mixed white and Amerindian ancestry) 30%; Aymara 25%; white 15%

3 Socioeconomic factors:
GDP per capita (International $)[c]   2568 (2002)
Health expenditure per capita (International $)[c]   179 (2002)
Health expenditure per GDP[c]   7.0% (2002)
Main industry[b,i]   Natural gas, mining (zinc, gold, silver, lead, tin, antimony); smelting; petroleum; soyabeans; food and beverages; tobacco; handicrafts; clothing; timber

4 Health factors:
Life expectancy at birth[c]   65.0 (M 63.0/F 67.0) (2003)
Five main causes of death[j]   Diseases of circulatory system, 30.3%; communicable diseases, 12.0%; external causes, 10.7%; neoplasms, 8.7%; conditions originating in the perinatal period, 5.4% (2000, ICD 10 used, coverage rate ≤ 63%)

5 Organisational factors:
Primary care model   Tripartite shared management model, 'DILOS', composed of representatives from the Ministry of Health and Sports (via the Departmental Health Services 'SEDES'), municipality and community (including indigenous peoples organisations and Oversight Committees); administrative and supervising roles by nurses; mobile health brigades (BRISAS) and ASISTES (community health agents) outreach the disadvantaged areas

Resources (health personnel)[e]	7.6 physicians/10 000 pop. (2001); 3.2 nurses and midwives/10 000 pop. (2001)
Financing[k]	National taxation; government budgets (prefecture, municipality); Productive and Social Investment Fund (FPS); National Solidarity Fund derived from the National Dialogue 2000 Special Account (HIPC II debt relief); Bolivian Social Security funds; private insurance funds; out-of-pocket payments; NGOs; international donations
Lead primary care practitioners	Auxiliary nurses and ASISTES

Policy priorities[m]

A *Equity, interculturality, and 'access and bridge'*
  Outreaching poor marginal areas through BRISAS and ASISTES in the EXTENSA programme; Universal Maternal and Child Health Insurance scheme (SUMI) (2003–) aims to enhance the demands of primary healthcare for mothers, and children aged under 5, as part of the Bolivian Poverty Reduction Strategy (EBRP); integrating traditional medicine providers into the formal health system

B *Decentralisation and participation based on the Popular Participation and Administrative Decentralisation Laws (1994/5)*
  New local health management model (local health committees, 'DILOS', and health networks of health establishments); shared local decision-making mechanism (e.g. Local Health Plans) through DILOS (possible NGO involvement in this process since 2002); national government ear-marked fund to municipalities (20%) and 10% assigned to the SUMI as the Popular Participation funds; municipalities are responsible for financing infrastructure and equipment with social control via community Oversight Committees; authority of the recruitment on human resources transferred to the department level

C *Management*
  Performance management through Information Analysis Committee (CAI) at multiple levels (e.g. CAI at the health establishment level involves community); conducting census on NGOs registered with the Ministry of Foreign Affairs, and establishing the tools for frameworks to monitor them; monitoring of municipal management at department (SEDES) and national levels

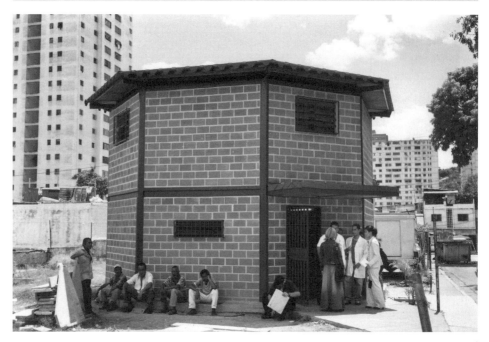

Figure 13   Caracas, Venezuela.

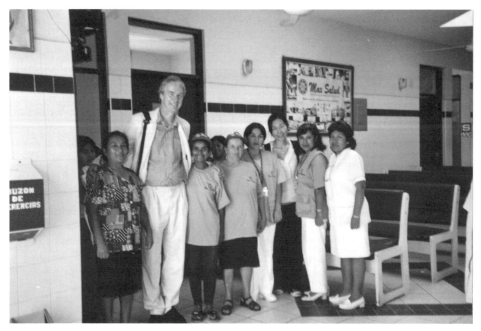

Figure 14   Chiclayo, Peru.

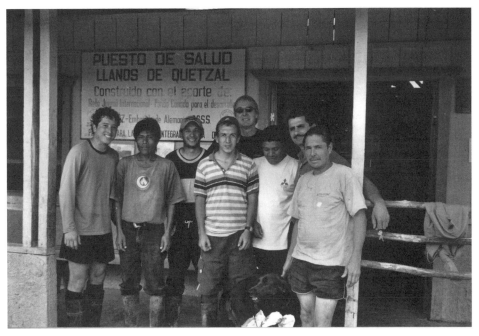

Figure 15   Community Development Agency, Costa Rica.

Figures 13–15 The community development agency (Venezuela, Peru, Costa Rica). The most exciting form of modern primary care organisation produces the most vivid images. In turn these are the unmistakable fortified *Consultorio Popular* new building in Caracas with its Cuban doctor in attendance. The blue t-shirted all-age volunteers at one of the *Chiclayo MaxSalud* health centres in Peru stand alongside Michiyo Iwami and Professor Meads; and the peripatetic primary care team at a Costa Rican *ebais* in the Chiclayo region. From left to right, they comprise a general medical practitioner, a healthcare technician, a community nurse, a dispenser, a medical records officer, a district administrator and a teacher. Four of these are indigenous people, locally recruited and trained.

Future prospects

In terms of its relationships for intensity and commitment, the model of the community development agency in primary care is unrivalled. Only the general practice comes even close. Relationships with the public; with a sometimes bewildering range of new partners as our exemplars in Costa Rica and Chiclayo especially illustrate; and with patients who feel they actually own the health-care practice themselves, are especially strong. As the Venezuelan and, to a lesser extent, Bolivian experiences demonstrate, policy makers can deploy this form of development for the purposes of cultural reconstruction at both local and national levels.

But, because of its grassroots power and origins, this is also the form of organisation that can generate the most enemies. Its relational dividends in the long term, after early bursts of enthusiasm at the inception of new service delivery units, are of mixed value. Unless they are willing to be authoritarian to the point of excess, policy makers lose control. Many professions are not only marginalised, but undervalued to the point of stigma. Their legitimate representatives, as well as elected politicians and independent academic experts, as in Caracas, can easily feel threatened by those with partisan interests and religious doctrines, who seek to usurp normal democratic processes by 'colonising' the leadership of community development initiatives and their vulnerable and often poorly educated participants.

Equity is a major dilemma with inequalities of health and resource status almost endemic to the nationwide system, notwithstanding attempts to ensure a fair and even distribution of logistics as in the San José approach to shared and modern information systems. So too is capacity. Venezuela remains dependent on 'dodgy deals' regarding Cuban imports. Bolivia is a model of legislative architecture not actions. In Peru the CLAS successes cannot disguise the need for the Ministry of Health to still manage most of the country's healthcare either directly or through historically established institutions, notwithstanding their deficiencies and secondary care bias.

Nevertheless, the community development agency is compatible with the Alma Ata principles of primary healthcare and to be commended accordingly. Its development is also compatible with that of many civil societies in relatively immature nation states (and sometimes their constituent parts) around the world. As such it may be seen as a staging post towards more mature modernised health systems, but given the political uncertainties in so many countries, it seems likely that for the present century at least it will be a prominent feature of the global primary care landscape.

References

1 Goecoechea J (ed.) (1996) *Primary Health Care Reforms*. Copenhagen: WHO.
2 Straten G, Friele K, Groenewegen P (2002) Public trust in Dutch health care. *Social Science and Medicine*. **55**: 227–34.
3 Son A (1999) Modernization of medical care in Korea. *Social Science and Medicine*. **49**: 543–50.
4 Meads G, Iwami M (2003) Latin lessons give a grassroots insight. *Primary Care Report*. **5**(2): 17–20.
5 Ministry of Health (2000) *Shared Administration Programme Direction*. Lima: MINSA.
6 Waters H, Abdallah H, Santillan D (2001) Application of activity-based costing for Peruvian NGO healthcare providers. *International Journal of Health Planning and Management*. **16**(1): 3–18.
7 Cotlear D, Sol Concha M, Castañeda T et al. (1999) *Peru: improving health care for the poor*. Washington, DC: World Bank.
8 Iwami M, Petchey R (2002) A CLAS act? Community-based organisations, health service decentralisation and primary care development in Peru. *Journal of Public Health Medicine*. **24**(4): 246–51.
9 Zuckerman E, de Kadt E (eds) (1997) *The Public-Private Mix in Social Services: health care and education in Chile, Costa Rica and Venezuela*. Washington, DC: Inter-American Development Bank.
10 Kahssay H, Oakley P (eds) (1999) *Community Involvement in Health and Development: a review of the concept and practice*. Geneva: WHO.

11 De Kadt E (2002) *Assessing Public-Private Approaches to Social Service Provision in Latin America: mixed experiences.* University of Utrecht: Department of Cultural Anthropology.
12 Pan American Health Organization (2002) *Health in the Americas: Bolivia,* vol. II. Washington, DC: Pan American Health Organization, pp.85–97.

Country profile sources

Peru, Costa Rica, Venezuela and Bolivia

a Population Division of the Department of Economic and Social Affairs of the United Nations Secretariat (2005) World Population Prospects: the 2004 revision population database. http://esa.un.org/unpp/ (accessed 22/06/05).
b Central Intelligence Agency (2005) The World Factbook. www.cia.gov (accessed 27/06/05).
c World Health Organization (2005) Core Health Indicators, WHO Statistical Information System. www.who.int (accessed 23/06/05).
d Pan American Health Organization (2003) *Health Statistics from the Americas.* Washington, DC: Pan American Health Organization.
e World Health Organization (2005) World Health Statistics 2005, WHO Statistical Information System. www.who.int (accessed 23/06/05).
f Adapted from World Health Organization (2005) WHO mortality database. www.who.int (accessed 08/09/05).
g Pan American Health Organization (2002) *Health in the Americas: Costa Rica,* vol. II. Washington, DC: Pan American Health Organization, pp.183–97.
h Pan American Health Organization (2002) Venezuela: health situation analysis and trends summary. www.paho.org (accessed 25/08/05).
i BBC (2005) BBC News Country Profile: Bolivia. http://news.bbc.co.uk (accessed 27/06/05).
j Pan American Health Organization (2002) *Health in the Americas: Bolivia,* vol. II. Washington, DC: Pan American Health Organization, pp.85–97.
k Cárdenas M (2004) *Health Sector Funding and Expenditure Accounts* (2e). La Paz: Ministerío de Salud y Deportes and DFID Bolivia; Washington, DC: World Bank; Washington, DC: Pan American Health Organization.
m The World Bank (2004) *Health Sector Reform in Bolivia: a decentralization case study.* Washington, DC: World Bank.

Chapter 8

The outreach franchise

Introduction

This organisational development for 'modernising' primary care is qualitatively distinct from the five described and illustrated in the preceding chapters. Where primary care is an outreach function and the object of alternative forms of subcontracting, it is not, almost by definition, part of the principal purpose of the public service commissioning agency and its main providers. In such situations a combination of resource limitations, cultural constraints and political dogma usually dictate that a national health system is essentially a hospital system. Primary care is designated by governments and with different degrees of design or default, as the responsibility of significant others. These may include charities, companies, councils, churches and communities themselves, with hospitals being the most common contractor and privatisation a frequent *motif* in attempts to establish effective and enduring franchise mechanisms. With outreach franchises an international analysis of the organisation of community services reveals wide differences in both management and clinical profiles. Few coherent patterns are apparent and the individual organisation within a particular country may well be both haphazard and *ad hoc*.

Without a unified or powerful payer the organisation of this model of primary care is, therefore, often variable and fragmented. At best, the network arrangements for sharing information and coordinating developments of a virtual organisation may apply,[1] with a few overarching aims and informal relationships creating links across a dispersed healthcare environment. Equity and consistent quality are invariably major issues of policy and practice. And public accountability is often in short supply. Family medicine itself is often reduced to no more than the small individual private practice, if it exists at all. But, notwithstanding these deficits and reservations, the outreach approach has advocates in abundance, many of whom are based in the world's fastest-growing economic locations. Cheap, contemporary, capitalist and controllable, franchising is their favoured response and 'solution' to almost any intractable issue, including health systems development.

Manila

'Smokey Mountain' is the popular description for the impoverished Manila suburbs of Tondo, teeming with a million-plus people, overcrowded 'Jeepney' buses and their graffiti-style murals and prefab shacks. The term stems from the piles of debris and domestic rubbish, smouldering continuously, we were told in 2004, since the end of the Second World War.

Only a short Jeepney ride away is Quezon City, the commercial centre of Manila where many international banks and businesses have their headquarters in The Philippines. Modern shopping malls proliferate. One of the newest is the Ortega Medical Plaza, a soaring tower block next to high-class tourist hotels and full of the widest range of private specialists' surgeries, laboratories, health insurance and pharmaceutical companies, and alternative therapy clinics. A high-level walkway traverses the highway linking the Medical Plaza to the main university hospital.

In Manila, primary care organisations have many faces. At Tondo, the local Aurora Health Centre, for example, relies on a motorbike and sidecar for most of its ambulance services. This vehicle weaves its way down narrow alleys, passageways and unmade streets. At the Quezon Medical Plaza there is swipe-card admission and heavily armed security. In The Philippines the policy for the franchising of primary care is unequivocally that of privatisation. At the time of our study in 2003/04 there were 30 designated national health programmes, but only six had significant government budgets. The status of primary care is indicated by the location of its responsible central policy makers in spartan Ministry of Health basement offices without windows. The main Department of General Practice in the country is similarly located in cramped conditions at The Philippines General Hospital, and across the country there are only a dozen officially accredited PhilHealth primary care centres.

Of the 600 working family physicians almost two-thirds are in full-time private practice. Historically the State Medicare scheme has offered only hospital insurance cover, and the policy objective of the Academy of Family Physicians of a 1:10 000 ratio in GP:patient relationships remains a distant aspiration. In Tondo, for instance, we found that the medical services for the 113 000 people covered by the BO Fuguso Health Centre are provided by just a socially conscientious paediatrician and a trainee family physician with six qualified nurses in support. Each morning a hundred-plus people wait outside for opening time in the hope of a consultation. They include many heavily pregnant women. Amidst the cases of pneumonia, tuberculosis, respiratory diseases and malnutrition, safe childbirth is a top priority and the BO Fugoso Centre's eight beds may all be used for 24 hours' 'lying-in'. Community health volunteers appointed by the Barangay Council in each subdistrict scour their designated 5–6000 populations for those close to delivery and local mayors campaign every three years for election on child health manifestos which closely reflect the country's overwhelming Roman Catholic religious affiliations.

In such a social context and political climate the organisation of primary care is often left to private initiatives and the socially conscientious. The promise of the proceeds from a minimal capitation payment and 3% payroll tax has to be seen as enough for a national government lacking both authority and resources, in the discharge of its national responsibilities for frontline public health and healthcare. In the words of one senior director interviewed at The Philippine Institute for Development Studies, 'alternative systems sprout', with non-governmental organisations and new donors particularly prominent. Those patients who can afford to, shop around, while in poorer areas like Tondo, municipal authorities are desperate for new payers and partners. The Lions and

Rotary Clubs, Marie Stopes and the Bayan Muna socialists are just some of the better-known contributors here to such 'community-based health development' as the Aurora and BO Fugosa Health Centres. These are registered with the national Council for Health and Development (CHD), which is also located in Quezon City. This seeks to provide training and evaluation programmes to non-statutory primary care organisations across The Philippines. Its funds frequently come from corporate and international sources including Japan and USAID, with Pfizer's generous 'Leaders in Health' programme being the most prominent recent attempt to protect and promote primary care professionals in rural areas.

The overall sense of this approach to outreach franchising is one of fragmentation and not a little frenzy. Overall trends and patterns are hard, if not impossible, to detect. Many doctors retrain as nurses and emigrate. The CHD has attempted to pull together the disparate endeavours into what a British Council interviewee called the 'complimentarism' required for 'a people's movement for growth'. But it has struggled, as has the Academy of Family Physicians in promulgating the set of 60 clinical guidelines it issued in 2003, to complement the CHD's requirements for registered providers to undertake 'community diagnosis' as the first step towards effective primary care.

Nevertheless, privatisation has brought some benefits. Nationally, some of the country's 80 health insurance companies, under pressure from PhilHealth, are now promoting a form of gatekeeping general practice. The *Tacloban* career ladder enables midwives, nurse practitioners and even Barangay health assistants to progress and train as family physicians. Across the country there are now 40 training units for this purpose. The expanded 53 Chapters of the Academy of Family Physicians now have 7500 members, with many former specialists seeing general practice as the future. Even in Tondo the local health centres are now enjoying training placements and volunteer attachments from those previously only practising their medicine in secondary care. As a 20% proportion of total healthcare expenditure the municipal levy for healthcare in Manila has now matched the central contribution and the new monies are almost entirely committed to community-based services. At first sight the apparently *laissez-faire* Filipino approach seems as dangerous to public health as are the streets of its capital city. These are almost without global parallel in terms of risk. On further investigation, however, the Sense of Place dictum[2] does apply to the privatisation of primary care. Outreach franchising fits The Philippines. There may be method in the Manila madness after all.

The Philippines

1 Capital city: Manila

2 Demographic factors:
Population size (million)[a]	83.05 (2005)
Age profile[a]	11.9% (aged < 5), 3.9% (aged 65 and over) (2005)
Ethnicity[b]	Christian Malay 91.5%; Muslim Malay 4%; Chinese 1.5%; other 3%

3 Socioeconomic factors:
GDP per capita (International $)[c]	5231 (2002)
Health expenditure per capita (International $)[c]	153 (2002)
Health expenditure per GDP[c]	2.9% (2002)
Main industry[b]	Electronics assembly; garments; footwear; pharmaceuticals; chemicals; wood products; food processing; petroleum refining; fishing

4 Health factors:
Life expectancy at birth[c]	68.0 (M 65.0/F 71.0) (2003)
Five main causes of death (rate per 100 000 population)[d]	Diseases of circulatory system, 133.53; diseases of respiratory system, 76.90; infectious and parasitic diseases, 65.95; external causes, 56.36; neoplasms, 44.03 (1998, ICD 9 BTL used, coverage rate 85.0%)

5 Organisational factors:
Primary care model	Private clinics, hospital outpatients or health management organisations (HMOs) in urban areas; municipal managed primary care, including public health at rural health units (RHUs) and Barangay health stations (BHSs) elsewhere
Resources (health personnel)[e]	11.6 physicians/10 000 pop. (2002); 61.4 nurses and midwives/10 000 pop. (2002)
Financing[f]	Out-of-pocket payments; government tax subsidies (national and local); employer and employee contributions (as well as indigent

informal sector premiums) for National Health Insurance Programme (NHIP); voluntary private health insurance funds; HMOs funds; external loans and donors

Lead primary care practitioners — Midwives and Barangay health workers (BHWs) in rural areas; GPs and nurses in urban areas

Policy priorities[g]

A *Protection*

Expanding the new NHIP coverage providing regular health screening programmes and primary healthcare services

B *Financing*

Adoption of capitation payments in healthcare financing for the local government units (LGUs)-led indigent programme in urban areas; cost-sharing between local authorities to support equitable healthcare

C *Partnership and participation*

Strengthen NGOs involvement in the local health boards (LHBs) with inter-sectoral approach to health (e.g. housing, education)

D *Management*

Cross-sectoral standards of licensing for healthcare providers by Philippine Health Insurance Corporation (PhilHealth); promoting incentive mechanisms (through partnership with local government units (LGUs)) including national quality assurance, the '*Sentrong Sigla'* movement; introduction of registered lists for insurance programmes to encourage effective referral services

E *Human resources*

Shifting to two-year volunteer community service placements for postgraduates from compulsory programme; family medicine conversion programmes for specialists via nationwide training units

Medan

The profile of healthcare provision in the town of Medan on the largest Indonesian island of Sumatra tells its own story. There are seven clinics and eight hospitals for a population in excess of two million. The former include two hospital-supported laboratories. The latter exclude the growing number of dedicated maternity units: a response to the high rate of abortions and pregnancy problems. These rank behind only intestinal infections in terms of hospital admissions across Indonesia. Although absent from the outdated national statistics, perinatal illnesses and poisoning are also often cited as major causes of mortality nationally and it is tempting in a country consisting of hot springs and vast plantations, and where there are so many islands that there are no reliable figures for their total, to employ geographic similes to describe the country's secondary care-dominated local health environments. A parallel with not only unplanned but unexplored jungles might be regarded as particularly apt.

To apply such terms would not be quite fair. Unlike in The Philippines, for example, the post-Sukarno presidential direction has not been simply to surrender to the non-governmental sector. There is a coherent nationwide framework of public administration for the contracting out or franchising of outreach services into communities. Notwithstanding its extraordinary cultural and linguistic mixtures – there are 583 different native tongues – the Indonesian legend for healthcare is *Bhinneka Tunggalika*: 'Unity in Diversity'. The Dutch colonial influence persists and, in Sumatra, seems to combine with a long cultural tradition of village *(Kepaladesa)* leaders and urban *(Kotomadya)* regents to sustain processes of civic order and organisation, which are headed by a governor. The mechanisms are in place for the effective receipt of and response to presidential instructions. As a Sukarno legacy, these are still often the favoured instrument for national policy implementation, with primary care coming under the auspices of the Ministry of Health and the People's Welfare Committee of the Indonesian House of Representatives. The latter has extended responsibilities for housing, social affairs and religious developments, as well as for public health.

Accordingly, in the Medan subdistrict administrators are agents of a centralised contracting process for primary care. At the time of our research (2003/04) they were responsible for ensuring the delivery of 16 basic local health services. These are, of course, not at all doctor dependent. The primary care model rather is a mix of mobile vehicles, including boats, community-designated health posts, and peripatetic nurses and midwives. The medical services of a doctor are accessed almost exclusively by coming into a town centre clinic or private hospital, the name of one of which in the Listrik neighbourhood nicely illustrates the Indonesian past and present: *Kumah Sakit Gleneagles*. Here is where the European doctors may still be found.

Complete and comprehensive cultural tolerance, with full religious freedoms, is a constitutional right in Indonesia. In Medan, as elsewhere, this *Pancasila* is also an absolute political necessity. Local institutional configurations, with their different powerful interest groups and histories, are untouchables. Hospitals are in this category. For primary care, franchising through local public administrative units recognises this unique scale and variety of community in Indonesia with central contracts for basic health services implemented in all sorts of ways with all sorts of practitioners. Healers and herbalists abound. For such issues as family planning, small grants to *Kepaladesa* and stipends for health information groups of 30-plus couples have gone further than might be expected in reducing birth rates and perinatal mortality.[3] The same applies to the inroads made on the control of respiratory diseases through the inclusion of environmental health in the central contracting process.

Medan, and Indonesia, defy the strategic logic of rational planning. But, after a fashion, and with the reinforcement of an authoritarian political culture, their franchises for the organisation of primary care work. Unlike in the other exemplars of this chapter they are designed not so much to promote privatisation but rather to be in parallel with it.

Indonesia

1 Capital city: Jakarta

2 Demographic factors:
  Population size (million)[a]   222.78 (2005)
  Age profile[a]   9.7% (aged < 5), 5.5% (aged 65 and
                                         over) (2005)
  Ethnicity[b]   Javanese 45%; Sundanese 14%;
                                         Madurese 7.5%; Coastal Malays
                                         7.5%; other 26%

3 Socioeconomic factors:
  GDP per capita (International $)[c]   3390 (2002)
  Health expenditure per capita
  (International $)[c]   110 (2002)
  Health expenditure per GDP[c]   3.2% (2002)
  Main industry[b]   Petroleum and natural gas; textiles,
                                         apparel, footwear; mining; cement
                                         chemical fertilisers; plywood;
                                         rubber; food; tourism

4 Health factors:
  Life expectancy at birth[c]   67.0 (M 65.0/F 68.0) (2003)
  Five known main causes of death[h]   Cardiovascular diseases; respiratory
                                         diseases; tuberculosis; infectious and
                                         parasitic diseases; diarrhoea (1995,
                                         figures are not available, coverage
                                         rate is not defined)

5 Organisational factors:
  Primary care model   Fixed and mobile doctor-led health
                                         centres serving as hubs to the
                                         nurse-led local subhealth centres;
                                         community managed family health
                                         posts with midwife and traditional
                                         healers at the village level
  Resources (health personnel)[e]   1.1 physicians/10 000 pop. (1998);
                                         4.9 nurses and midwives/10 000
                                         pop. (2000)
  Financing[i]   National government subsidies and
                                         ear-marked revenues; government
                                         revenues (regional and local); out-
                                         of-pocket payments; employer-
                                         sponsored health benefits for
                                         employees; private health insurance
                                         funds; community health insurance
                                         schemes; external loans and grants
  Lead primary care practitioners   Nurses

Policy priorities[j]

A *Health education and promotion (HEP)*
  KAP (knowledge, attitude and practice) approach to promoting public health at family and community levels that aims to improve environmental health, food and the lifestyles of the population

B *Fair financing*
  Developing equitable national health insurance schemes; adjustment in payment of care services for the poor at private health facilities to ensure equal access

C *Participation*
  Facilitating bottom-up planning mechanisms via development coordination/consultation meetings at different levels which embrace environmental health within the development agenda; strengthen involvement of NGOs and public in implementation of national health programmes (e.g. HIV/AIDS control, maternal and child health, etc.), and local volunteer workers

Tokushima

All of our interviewees in Japan were agreed on one thing: Japan does not really 'do' primary care. The Japanese Society of Primary Care may date back to 1978 and there is a small Academy of Primary Care Physicians in Tokyo, but overwhelmingly this is a national system based on state-sponsored public health, social insurance-driven care management and large-scale acute sector hospital provision. The concept of the GP in both medicine and nursing is absent. There are no gatekeepers, exclusive personal medical lists, multiprofessional teams or practice nurses. Capitation payment mechanisms are eschewed and the notion of social medicine undertaken from community settings is an anathema to the bewildering combination of overlapping insurers and providers for whom the protection of fee for service arrangements is both a reciprocal self-interest and a historic duty.

There are over 3300 municipalities in Japan and, accordingly, at the Tokushima *hoken* (public health) centre we found no doctors. With the same total establishment of 37 personnel as the Wimborne extended general practice described in Chapter 3, its professional profile could scarcely be more different. There are 27 fully qualified public health nurses, plus two nursing assistants. Half of these focus exclusively on maternal and child health. The remaining staff are a dental hygienist, administrators and a managing nutritionist. Theirs is what they term a 'total (i.e. comprehensive) approach'. Operating to the terms of the 2003 Health Promotion Law and the latest national new 'Gold Plan', its programmes each look to have a three-pronged impact on *Kokoro* (mind), *Kurashi* (lifestyle) and *Karada* (body). The sequence is significant. It is the reverse order to most Western countries. Health improvement is a way of thinking first and then a way of being and behaving. This is an approach that has historically taken Japan to the top of global league tables for life expectancy with its post-wartime emphasis on prevention and early disease detection.

Major attempts at health service reorganisation have historically been eschewed in favour of 'muddling through'.[4] This has meant high costs in terms of overall financial cost and professional power. Japan, for example, has the highest number of computed tomography (CT) and magnetic resonance imaging (MRI) scanners in the world. But it is also world famous for its low levels of social deviance in terms of crime, drugs, poverty, diet, divorce rates and welfare.

Health checks in Japan are frequent and mandatory: at annual intervals, for example, after the age of 40, with dementia a specific screening target. Facilities are first class in the Tokushima centre: a gymnasium, a public bath, parentcraft and publications, a battery of freely available tests for *inter alia* hypertension, HIV and heart disease; and designated 'Health Mates' for those targeted as overweight. Excellent sanitation and dietary standards are actively promoted and monitored as part of National Nutrition Programme arrangements, which had their first annual report as far back as 1951.

Moreover, at this centre there are facilities to call on a paediatrician and three generalist doctors and a dentist from a neighbouring municipal clinic. In child protection and emergency night-time cases, in particular, this is helpful. It is also unusual. The norm is hospital outpatient attendance or an appointment with a private *Kakaritsukei* or *Shujii*. These are 'specialoids': specialists offering supplementary general services. By definition the Japanese words prescribed by the National Medical Association preclude a single personal doctor–patient relationship and entitle the citizen to a choice of specialoids. That Tokushima is able to establish and manage a small medical centre with something akin to family doctors is entirely because of its population size as a city of 270 000. At 300 000 all responsibilities for medical care pass to the prefecture, of which there are 47 in Japan. Almost invariably, as in adjacent Osaka, this means that all the *hokenjo* (medical care) managed by municipalities has been brought together at a single hospital-based site with, at best, its own primary care clinics and peripatetic facilities.

It also means, across prefectures, different rates of charging for municipal-level extensions to *hokenjo*. In Tokushima, outpatient medical care is free only for the first two years. Next door in Kagawa it is free for all pre-school age children. The Tokushima localised model is more expensive and, although nationally most screening tests are free, since the introduction of universal medical coverage through the National Health Insurance Act in 1961 all Japanese people have become accustomed to accessing a doctor for a specific service in respect of a specific condition for a specific charge covered by a premium payment and, where required, a co-contribution. Even the municipalities exercise their public health responsibilities through taxation funding raised in the form of local insurance schemes.

It is the particular and complex framework of insurance which ultimately determines the outreach franchises for primary care beyond *hokenjo* even in Tokushima. Over 13 000 different medical procedures are covered as insured items. There are more than 3400 independent health insurance plans across Japan. They are of several different types and are expanding, especially since the introduction of compulsory long-term social care insurance and care management in 2000. For example, in addition to the government's national insurance scheme for retired and self-employed people and their dependants, there are two classes of employees' medical insurance. There are also two types of payment under the new long-term care insurance arrangements for those over 40 and those over 65. For the former, the 50% employee and employer contributions, reductions against medical insurance premiums, and growing levels of co-payments required for residential and inpatient care have meant that gradually Japanese people are becoming more proactive in negotiating their own care packages. The government sets national fee schedules and regulates payer prices across the country. Gradually too, as part of its Healthy Japan 21 initiatives,[5] it is using these mechanisms to promote clinic attendance away from hospitals, generic drug usage and the inclusion of *Katei Gakkou* (family and school) doctors in preferential premiums. Many of these medical professionals remain based in private hospitals.

The overall result is an increase of 17 000 in the number of provider options by 2003 and the further development of community mutual aid societies. Nationally there are over 34 000 care managers and past patient passivity is slowly giving way as insurance cover contracts shift their orientation from *Sochi* (supply side) to *Keiyaku* (user negotiation). In the universities, the restrictions of controlling consultant-led *Ikyoku* education groupings in hospitals are beginning to be addressed by proposals for a new two-year primary care post-qualifying medical qualification. In Tokushima, the family doctors we met talked of moving to 'a personalised health service from a food and property health service'. They looked to local housewives to champion their cause and Chiba University for the necessary curricula.

Nevertheless, there is a long way to go before Japan can claim its own authentic organisational developments in primary care. Politically the latter remains part of the Ministry of Labour and Welfare. Public health status is an economic and employment prerequisite and medicine remains the property of specialists in hospitals, four out of five of which are in the private sector, publicly funded and profit making through the plethora of different premiums and payment mechanisms. Even in Tokushima it is the agents of insurance that shape the configuration for outreach healthcare and the franchising for 'specialoid' services.

Japan	
1 Capital city:	Tokyo
2 Demographic factors:	
Population size (million)[a]	128.09 (2005)
Age profile[a]	4.6% (aged < 5), 19.7% (aged 65 and over) (2005)
Ethnicity[b]	Japanese 99%; others 1% (Korean 511 262, Chinese 244 241, Brazilian 182 232, Filipino 89 851, other 237 914)

3 Socioeconomic factors:
   GDP per capita (International $)[k] 26 860 (2002)
   Health expenditure per capita
   (International $)[k]   2133 (2002)
   Health expenditure per GDP[k]   7.9% (2002)
   Main industry[b]   Motor vehicles; electronic equip-
                                          ment; machine tools; steel and
                                          nonferrous metals; ships; chemicals;
                                          textiles; processed foods

4 Health factors:
   Life expectancy at birth[k]   81.5 (M 78.0/F 85.0) (2003)
   Five main causes of death
   (rate per 100 000 population)[d]   Neoplasms, 249.11; diseases of
                                          circulatory system, 240.53; diseases
                                          of respiratory system, 108.64; exter-
                                          nal causes, 90.29; diseases of diges-
                                          tive system, 30.52 (2002, ICD 10
                                          used, coverage rate 100%)

5 Organisational factors:
   Primary care model   Doctors at privately founded clinics
                                          working as independent entrepre-
                                          neurs with mostly solo practice;
                                          hospital outpatient services; and
                                          preventive and promotive services
                                          (e.g. food, sanitation) at public
                                          health centres
   Resources (health personnel)[e]   20.1 physicians/10 000 pop. (2000);
                                          86.3 nurses and midwives/10 000
                                          pop. (2000)
   Financing[m]   Employers and employees contribu-
                                          tions (premiums) for multiple
                                          compulsory social insurance
                                          schemes according to age, employ-
                                          ment status, and locations; taxation
                                          (national, prefectural, local);
                                          government subsidies; out-of-pocket
                                          payments; private health insurance
                                          funds
   Lead primary care practitioners[n]   'Specialoids'

Policy priorities[m,o,p]
A *Health promotion*
   Through Health Promotion Law (2002) services operated by prefectures and municipalities at public health centres; 'Healthy Japan 21'
   ten-year programme promotes good health and happy living through
   changing behaviours, promoting early screening programmes

B *Financing*
Strict cost control system for national fee schedules and pricing of drugs and DRG procedures

C *Long-term care insurance (LTCI) (2000–)*
For the elderly and senile, encourages them to live independently in their own homes

D *Partnership and participation*
Involvement of private care providers in LTCI scheme, including non-profit organisations (NPOs) and commercial companies, to widen choice for users and flexibility in the market; promoting user involvement in decision making of care plans with care managers in LTCI

E *Human resources*
Two-year minimum new compulsory training programmes for post-graduates (2004–) focusing on primary care and interpersonal skills

F *Management*
Risk management through pooling insurance premiums at prefecture level, redistributing them to municipalities according to demographics and income level, and joint management programmes; 'Healthy Japan 21' programme set goals by 2010 in nine areas including nutrition, exercise, smoking, relaxation and mental health

Shanghai

The three forms of contracting out so far described in this chapter are not organisational development options for primary care in China. It cannot turn to the private markets, municipal administrations or insurance agencies available in, respectively, The Philippines, Indonesia and Japan. Despite recent democratisation, its only viable option for franchising remained the commune, at the time of our visit.

Shanghai, like China itself, is formidably institutional in its public service structures. Community health attracts less than 1% of its public healthcare expenditure. Across the country there are 10 000 secondary and tertiary care hospitals and 100 000-plus special needs hospitals for older and infirm citizens, disabled and mentally ill people. The 14 million population of Shanghai has its full share of both types of institution, which total 590 in all. These include ten national specialist centres and 30 Grade One acute hospitals: more than two for each of the city's 13 districts.

The Putuoqu Hospital in the Putau district is one of these with over 800 beds and 1250 staff, including 400 doctors. None of these work in the community. But they do provide 860 000 outpatient sessions a year. People queue from before dawn to attend. They pay between three and five *yuan* depending on the consultant. Some can reclaim from their employers. About a fifth attend for traditional Chinese medicine therapies, including people who are diabetics, asthmatics and stroke victims. The latter especially favour the technique of acupuncture. There are specialist private practices in the district. They are almost invariably run by dentists. Sometimes a doctor does do a domiciliary visit in problematic postnatal cases, but this is the exception rather than the rule. Usually they are left to the barefoot doctors to deal with, especially in the rural areas, or to whatever support communally can be garnered through the local party members' neighbourhood committee.

In the district of Shanghai we visited, such support amounts to another hospital with 80 beds but no resident doctors, only nurses. Some of these are trained at accredited medical colleges. Some are not. State registration comes after three years, the same period that should apply for rural medicine. Many barefoot doctors, however, have received only a rudimentary three-month period of supervised induction for their roles. They practise from the most basic of surgery facilities with minimal drug stores augmented by a huge range of herbal and natural remedies. There are no operating theatres at the neighbourhood hospital, just a minor casualty unit and maintenance facilities. For most conditions, and anything serious, the patient has to go to Putuoqu.

The neighbourhood committee does what it can. Lower in authority than the hospital president, in terms of Communist Party membership status, it has a kindergarten, schools, custodial units, and preferential access to jobs and apprenticeships. Past authoritarian lines of command operate to some effect to control birth rates, compulsory minimum ages for marriage and wider health promotion campaigns. In practice, both high-cost healthcare technologies and remote areas are entirely dependent on external charities, particularly after a prolonged period of substantial reductions in central government healthcare expenditure.[6] The inner cities are the political and economic priority, where citizens have new medical savings and social pooling accounts.[7] As a result, rural China is fertile territory now for international mission-based healthcare development. It fills a deliberate void. China, surprisingly, has the largest and fastest-growing number of Christian believers on the planet and a commensurate increase in evangelical literature.[8,9] T'ai chi before breakfast and Singapore-sponsored house church meetings in the evening are representative of the curious new Chinese cultural combinations[10] that place charities alongside communists in the franchised outreach arrangements for frontline healthcare.

There is, of course, a five-year National Health Plan. Decentralisation is central to this. So too is prevention. But planned public healthcare expenditure was only 3.5% of GDP when we interviewed government policy advisers at the Ministry of Health. They said they hoped to control the licensing of hospitals, as well as the birth rate and the spread of HIV infections. They also hoped to introduce general medical practitioners, so long as they are willing to be full-time State employees, not independent contractors. But the projected expenditure means only £20 per capita per annum, and most hospitals we visited were starved of government grants and heavily in debt. In government there is no resource, let alone the will, for a primary care organisation. It has to be left to others.

China

1 Capital city:	Beijing

2 Demographic factors:

Population size (million)[a]	1315.84 (2005)
Age profile[a]	6.4% (aged < 5), 7.6% (aged 65 and over) (2005)
Ethnicity[b]	Han Chinese 91.9%; Zhuang, Uygur, Hui, Yi, Tibetan, Miao, Manchu, Mongol, Buyi, Korean, and other nationalities 8.1%

3 Socioeconomic factors:

GDP per capita (International $)[c]	4460 (2002)
Health expenditure per capita (International $)[c]	261 (2002)
Health expenditure per GDP[c]	5.8% (2002)
Main industry[b]	Mining and ore processing; iron, steel, aluminum and other metals; coal; machine building; armaments; textiles and apparel; petroleum; cement; chemicals; fertilisers; consumer products, including footwear, toys and electronics; food processing; transportation equipment, including automobiles, rail cars and locomotives, ships and aircraft; telecommunications equipment, commercial space launch vehicles and satellites

4 Health factors:

Life expectancy at birth[c]	71.0 (M 70.0/F 73.0) (2003)
Five main causes of death in urban areas (death rate per 100 000 population)[q]	Malignant neoplasms, 119.71; cerebrovascular diseases, 88.37; diseases of respiratory system, 78.06; heart diseases, 74.12; injury and poisoning, 43.45 (2002, coverage rate is not defined)

5 Organisational factors:

Primary care model	Hospital-based clinics and private practitioners in urban areas; village/township health centres and 'barefoot' doctors in rural areas with Chinese medicine practitioners
Resources (health personnel)[e]	16.4 physicians/10 000 pop. (2002); 9.6 nurses and midwives/10 000 pop. (2003)
Financing[q,r]	Out-of-pocket payments; contributions from the collective and voluntary household premiums and local government subsidies for Rural Cooperative Medical Systems (RCMS); urban employees basic medical insurance system funds government subsidies; funds from Medical Savings Accounts (social pooling accounts, individual savings accounts) for urban health insurance system; external loans
Lead primary care practitioners	Trainee doctors (rural) and specialist physicians (urban)

Policy priorities[r,s]

A *Management and regulation of mixed provision*
Combining healthcare schemes for cost control; rationalisation of hospital resources planned at regional level; developing the three-tier health network; financial support for rural primary healthcare; introduction of essential drug lists; shifting towards contract arrangements and performance-based recruitment of health personnel; separate accounting systems for prescribing and dispensing drugs; regulation of hospital sector (for-profit, not-for-profit); minimum period of rural community placement for the promotion of urban doctors

B *Equitable access to care and comprehensive primary healthcare*
Re-establishing the rural cooperative medical system (RCMS) with pilot projects based on Rural Health Policy (2001) through modernising basic equipment and health facilities, providing training programmes for health workers to improve professional competency, and management skills that aim to encourage utilisation of services and respond more effectively to the needs of the rural poor; focusing on public health and emergent diseases, including SARS, sexual health (HIV/AIDS, STIs) and tuberculosis control and prevention, through the Centre for Disease Prevention and Control, and epidemic prevention stations

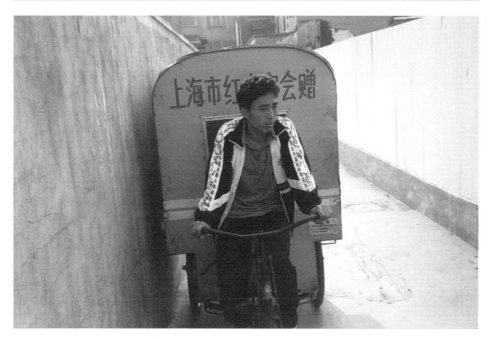

Figure 16   Shanghai, China.

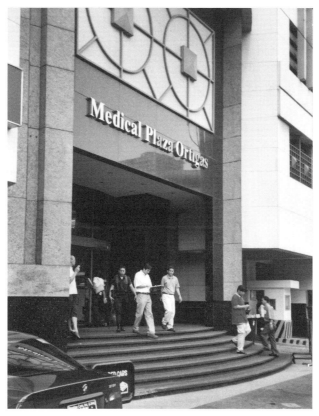

Figure 17   Philippines.

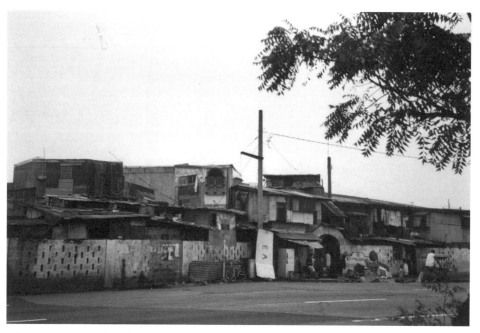

Figure 18   Tondo, Philippines.

Figures 16–18 Franchised outreach (China, Philippines, Philippines). The primitive level and widely varying status of primary care is illustrated by the two images of clinic transport and commercial facilities from Shanghai and Manila, with the final photograph showing a typical residential block in the latter's impoverished Tondo district.

Future prospects

The model of primary care described in this chapter is flourishing in a part of the world which, as a result of globalisation, is advancing rapidly in terms of economic growth and political influence. Its community health services reflect the prevalent East Asian philosophy: low cost and high-turnover production, inexpensive labour, unregulated and non-unionised, and consumer driven. It is a philosophy that in both economic and social policy terms can prove attractive elsewhere. It limits the burden on governments, prevents professional or corporate capture of health systems and can be promulgated through political messages emphasising personal responsibility and popular choice. As past studies have shown in Japan,[11] these can be successfully attached to a powerful and relatively inexpensive public health movement.

In respect of relationships the advance of franchised outreach primary care organisations, however, offers very mixed blessings. As our four exemplars illustrate, any benefits accrued in terms of our six categories for potential relationship dividends are likely to be, at best, localised and time limited. We have not come across any consistent intra- or interprofessional developments. As a policy priority, primary care is low and the consumerist orientation tends to diminish the rights and role of both patients individually and the public, through legitimate representative mechanisms in decision making.

The only area for an enhanced relationship dividend is that with new partners. The contracting out of primary care relies on others to respond and, if necessary, to replace past health service providers. There are large gaps to be filled, and whether for motives of profit, or more altruistically to pick up the pieces, novel collaborations are shaped. These bring with them new and additional ideas, energies and resources and, as in China and Indonesia, can gain such a positive communal response that local civic regeneration may occur. The problem remains, however, that even in the likes of Shanghai or Medan, it is not primary care that is the principal purpose of the new partners, whether they be mission agencies, local authorities or insurance companies. For all of them primary care is a means to another end. If the East Asian organisational model is to be a further technological export it seems important that such continental counterparts as the European Union ensure there are sufficient safeguards for the protection and preservation of their member countries' more relationally committed healthcare systems.

References

1 Meads G, Ashcroft J (2000) *Relationships in the NHS*. London: RSM Press, pp.62–3.
2 Hanlon N (2001) Sense of place: organizational context and the strategic management of publicly funded hospitals. *Health Policy*. **58**: 151–73.
3 Shiffman J (2002) The construction of community participation: village family planning groups and the Indonesian state. *Social Science and Medicine*. **54**: 1199–214
4 Ikegami N, Creighton Campbell J (1999) Health care reform in Japan: the virtues of muddling through. *Health Affairs*. **18**(3): 56–75.
5 Health Service Bureau (2003) *People's Health Promotion Campaign for the Twenty First Century*. Tokyo: Ministry of Health, Labour and Welfare.
6 Xingzhu Liu, Mills A (2000) Financing reforms of public health services in China. *Social Science and Medicine*. **54**: 1691–8.
7 Liu GG, Zhongyon Zhao, Ruhua Cai et al. (2002) Equity in health care access: assessing the urban health insurance reform in China. *Social Science and Medicine*. **55**: 1779–94.
8 Lambert T (1999) *China's Christian Millions*. London: Monarch Books.
9 Paterson R (1999) *The Continuing Heart Cry for China*. Tonbridge: Sovereign World.
10 Meads G (2004) Change in China: where now for primary care? *Primary Care Report*. **6**(13): 10–13.
11 Ohtaki J, Fujisaki K, Terasaki H et al. (1996) Specialty choice and understanding of primary care among Japanese medical students. *Medical Education*. **30**: 378–84.

Country profile sources

The Philippines, Indonesia, Japan and China

[a] Population Division of the Department of Economic and Social Affairs of the United Nations Secretariat (2005) World Population Prospects: the 2004 revision population database. http://esa.un.org/unpp/ (accessed 22/06/05).
[b] Central Intelligence Agency (2005) The World Factbook. www.cia.gov (accessed 27/06/05).

c   World Health Organization (2005) Core Health Indicators, WHO Statistical Information System. www.who.int (accessed 23/06/05).

d   Adapted from World Health Organization (2005) WHO mortality database. www.who.int (accessed 08/09/05).

e   World Health Organization (2005) World Health Statistics 2005, WHO Statistical Information System. www.who.int (accessed 23/06/05).

f   Ramirez MC (ed.) (1999) Health Sector Reform Agenda (HSRA) 1999–2004. HSRA Monograph series No. 2, DoH. www.doh.gov.ph (accessed 05/09/05).

g   Department of Health: The birth of *Sentrong Sigla*. www.doh.gov.ph (accessed 05/09/05).

h   WHO/SEARO. Five leading causes of mortality in the SEA Region, by country, 1994–2000. http://w3.whosea.org/eip/TAB43.htm (accessed 30/08/05).

i   World Health Organization (2004) Indonesia. www.who.int (accessed 09/09/05).

j   WHO/SEARO. Country Health Profile: Indonesia. http://w3.whosea.org/ (accessed 15/08/05).

k   World Health Organization (2005) Japan. www.who.int (accessed 23/06/05).

m   Ministry of Health, Labour and Welfare (2002) MHLW White Paper. Tokyo: MHLW.

n   Ikegami N (2002) The Japanese Health Care System – structure, dynamics, lessons. London: LSE seminar (presentation slides).

o   Ministry of Health, Labour and Welfare and Japan International Corporation of Welfare Services (2002) *The 12th Study Programme for the Asian Social Insurance Administrators*. Tokyo: MHLW and JICWELS.

p   Ministry of Health, Labour and Welfare. *Health Japan 21: Let's start together*. Tokyo: MHLW.

q   Regional Office for the Western Pacific, World Health Organization (2004) Country Health Information Profile: China. www.wpro.who.int (accessed 13/07/05).

r   Walford V (2000) *China: health briefing paper*. London: DFID Resource Centre for Health Sector Reform. www.dfidhealthrc.org/Shared/publications/Country_health /China.pdf#search='China%3A%20health%20briefing%20paper%20DFID%20Reso urce%20Centre%20for%20Health%20Sector%20Reform' (accessed 05/09/05).

s   Lin V, Zhao H (2001) Health policy and financing in China: an update for AusAID. www.latrobe.edu.au/publichealth/downloads/AusAID_HealthPolicyChina.pdf#searc h='China%20health%20financing (accessed 05/09/05).

Chapter 9

Transferable learning

Towards a new theory

In September 2005 I was asked to make a closing presentation on the subject of global developments in primary care to a wide-ranging audience of representatives from Mexican health services organisations.[1] As usual, I described and emphasised the diversity of organisational initiatives taking place. At the time I thought I was merely echoing the comments made by several of my fellow speakers from Argentina, Brazil, Canada, Israel, Spain and the US, who had each outlined recent changes within their particular national environments. But then one of the local hosts summed up our contributions. Of course, he complimented each of us, but when it came to my turn, he remarked rather dryly: 'According to Professor Meads the term "primary care" is virtually meaningless. It is no more and no less than whatever the first contact practitioner has to offer in any particular situation. There is no consistency at all.' It felt for a moment as though the lights had been turned off. Instead of some enlightenment, my international perspective seemed only to have brought with its myriad of different images, a blackening sense of confusion and *ennui*. That the same speaker then concluded that 'for all its flaws' the British health system 'led the world' seemed scant consolation.

I do hope that neither of these reactions is the experience of the readers of this book. While primary care is not as simple and one-dimensional as it often seemed in the twentieth century, there are nevertheless some consistent trends as well as individual highlights to be detected, and both offer opportunities to emulate and to excite at local levels in other settings. The many international moves towards multiple forms of financing and wider custodianship roles in community health and development, for example, have thrown up in the preceding chapters several instances of specific new initiatives with which we in the UK, at least, are not familiar. More generally, the simple basic trend across countries from Portugal to Thailand and Finland to Chile in the direction of 30 000 populations for the modern primary care organisation is a practical fact which policy makers everywhere would do well to take into account. The aggregate collected data does indicate that it is time to revisit and even revise, where necessary, some of the established ideas and concepts of primary care. There are identifiable overall trends and together these merit their own modern theories: to both explain the organisation and guide the practice of primary care.

In terms of past definitions of primary care, these tend to fall into three categories which a WHO policy adviser has recently characterised as the 'ideal', the 'operational' and the 'political'.[2] The first two have been the most numerous. As a result, definitions have tended to be values based and prescriptive rather than neutral and descriptive. They have stated what (in the writer's view) should happen. Conceptualising the actual practice of primary care in theoretical terms based on (objective) empirical research has tended not to be a task undertaken by academic contributors, with very few exceptions.[3]

The prescriptive nature of the definitions is evident in that provided below by Barbara Starfield in her authoritative revised text of 1998. It is the most frequently cited contemporary definition and runs as follows:

> *Primary care is that level of a health system that provides entry into the system for all new needs and problems, provides person-focused (not disease oriented) care over time, provides care for all but very uncommon or unusual conditions, and coordinates or integrates care provided elsewhere or by others.*[4] *(pp.8–9)*

This definition may be seen as in a line relationship with the WHO 1978 Alma Ata Declaration, which was the classic ideal statement. The extract that follows points to conditions of being never yet achieved in any national health system; and one that is never likely to exist. The 1978 Declaration asserted that primary health care should:

- Evolve from both the social and economic conditions of a country reflecting its cultural characteristics and communities through relevant social, biomedical and health services research.
- Address the main public health problems of a community, providing comprehensive promotive, preventive, curative and rehabilitative services.
- Involve all related sectors and aspects of national and community development in pursuit of public health for all.
- Require and promote community participation and individual self-reliance to underpin the planning, organisation and delivery of health services, maximising the available resources and the educational opportunities for public health improvement.
- Sustain integrated and mutually supportive referral systems with priority given to those most in need by health workers trained both socially and technically to operate as teams targeting priority groups.

Put together, the above and a list of required service functions meant that an optimal condition of spiritual, physical and mental wellbeing could be claimed as the outcome for primary healthcare.[5]

This was, indeed, a heady brew and subsequent definitions have been strongly influenced by this aspirational approach. The most recent WONCA statements, for example, have listed in one instance of over 48 pages, no fewer than 11 'central characteristics', six 'core competencies' and three essential 'background features' for every family doctor;[6] and ten basic attributes of primary care in the other.[7] The following table summarises these statements, illustrating how definitions derived from a partisan professional perspective incline towards the functional.

Table 9.1 Professional perspectives on primary care

WONCA (2002a)[6]	WONCA (2002b)[7]
1 Management of primary care contacts service coordination	1 Management of primary–secondary care interface
2 Person-centred longitudinal care	2 General physician services to a community
3 Comprehensive approach to health promotion and maintenance	3 Locality-based public health leadership
4 Problem solving to facilitate prevention and effective clinical interventions	4 Specialist service of clinical care, research and education
5 Community oriented to match needs and resources	5 Gateway to computerised information and advice
6 Holistic modelling to contextualise biomedical diagnoses and inputs	6 Partnership of equal contributions from local professions

Inevitably such functional definitions have been as dominated by general medical practitioners as those in 'ideal' mode have been by global public health agencies. Among the latter the growing influence of economic organisations has been more evident as the focus has shifted from primary care *per se* to poverty.[8] The WHO's own millennium statement[9] regarding the pre-conditions for primary healthcare, accordingly, introduced employment conditions for workers, local organisational capacity, and quality assurance and audit regimes to its shortlist of the functional requirements it would look to in future assessments of sustainable primary care reform programmes. These pre-conditions have led in turn to a series of methodological developments in terms of evaluating and monitoring primary care performance.[10,11] These apply equally now to both developing and developed countries and one of the consistent modern trends in primary care is its organisations' use of targetry and general management techniques.

Political definitions of primary care have been less popular. That primary care has long been a malleable term of political discourse, or what one commentator called 'a linguistic accommodation',[12] there can be little doubt. But political analyses have historically been identified either with comparatively marginal movements – such as that of community-oriented primary care[13,14] – or radical campaigning ideologies such as that which looks to highlight the dangers of primary care development becoming the vanguard vehicle for privatisation.[15,16] In short, politics and advocacy have gone together and become intertwined.

As a result, Barnard's political categorisation of primary care has been devalued.[2] In the post-millennium period this is not only unfortunate, it is also a major stumbling block for both policy makers and practitioners looking to further progress the cause of primary care development. For, as our case exemplars have demonstrated, the modern organisations of primary care are far more than culturally compliant and locally apposite. Invariably they are now deliberate cultural constructions that draw on international and intersectoral resources in their creation. No longer can they be understood as individual units of independent professionals, but rather as collective agencies that are part of complex and highly interactive organisational developments. The pattern of relationships in the primary care of the twenty-first century is fundamentally changing.

Yet what people are looking for in these relationships is not. Fundamentally it stays the same in terms of personal trust and care, over time and across the spectrum of life's issues and presenting problems. The political imperative for primary care is to ensure that these needs are met empathically by the modern pattern of relationships in primary care. From Venezuela to Thailand, from New Zealand to Costa Rica, the notion of the medical or nursing professional is not enough. Everywhere, through globalisation, that which people most hold dear are the soccer clubs such as Chelsea and Real Madrid with international sponsors, the global instant news broadcasting satellite channels, ethnic music and foreign cuisine, the clothing brand names of multinational corporations, borderless Internet communications and worldwide iconic symbols from Mother Teresa to Pope John Paul II and Princess Diana. In the UK the traditional local surgery unit of primary care is, politically, as antiquated and ripe for change as was the Rover (or even British Leyland) car manufacturer when it was an exclusively domestic product. In the primary care of the twenty-first century, the people everywhere will want to select and identify with their primary care supplier just as closely as they now do with their BMW, Toyota or Peugeot – whether it be brand new in the West or ten years old-plus in countries south of the Equator.

A political definition of primary care based on actual developments worldwide would include the following elements.

- The diversity of organisational developments (and the futility of arguing now for a single, standard model).
- The growth in both provider catchment area and mixed personnel, including non- and semi-professionals in the service unit.
- The network patterns of relationships both internally and externally.
- The formative impact of corporate entities on the organisation of primary care as integral to social and economic capital development.
- The tension between increasingly influential information-based communities and those based on geographic or demographic boundaries.
- The universal requirement for accountability through management and visible performance indicators and measures.
- The advent of alternative and often multiple funding sources and new stakeholders for whom primary care is a secondary investment not a principal commitment.
- The opportunity afforded by modern primary care developments for governments to seek to radically reform and revive direct and civic relationships with electorates bypassing professional and other established elites.
- The role of primary care in the twenty-first century in significantly influencing profiles of political power, particularly through its locations for knowledge management.

As the number and scale of each of the above indicate – especially the final listed element – contemporary primary care is now a subject to which we do a disservice if we stick solely to our more comfortable functional and idealist perspectives.

Towards a new practice

A footnote to finish, principally for those engaged in the practice of primary care, but also with some policy makers, especially in the UK, in mind. For both, there has been a danger in recent years of being so consumed with the operational overload of continuous and often cosmetic organisational changes that it has been hard to look over the parapets. Independent political study and analysis has often been eschewed, even by leading general medical practitioners[17] (and indeed the present author[18]) by blind adherence to one form of new primary care organisation. The desire has been to make it work. The outcome, however, has normally been no more than a slogan or a label for a short-term transitional phase.

The challenge for those engaged in primary care, therefore, is to be participant observers. Contemporary policy processes are more participative. They may be heading, through universally available impact assessments and their data, in the direction of a genuine 'public choice' model,[19] but they also remain profoundly institutional in their vertical tiers of decision making and controls. Political participation in the organisational developments described in the previous chapters and analysed earlier in the present one, has still to be conditional. The criteria for involvement must be that of additional relationships value – to the health of communities and the healthcare of individuals – particularly when so many of the influences impinging on modern primary care organisations are so powerfully economic and ideological, even if sometimes they are marketed in ways that might not make them seem so.

During the last century the new bureaucracies of governments seeking to establish public service structures such as that of the National Health Service in England gradually learnt that institutional approaches were more effective when they become more incremental in their implementation and even formulation of major policies.[20] Perhaps the same lesson now needs to be learnt again, but this time especially by practitioners. Incremental primary care development requires more negotiation, over time and through reflection. It can mean some participants sometimes saying 'No', and always means more participants, eventually, saying 'Yes'. The behavioural choice is not just to either compete or collaborate, but also to critique and even confront. More haste and less speed is the Scandinavian style where international primary care at the start of the twenty-first century is best. As the next millennium proceeds, perhaps this is a lesson for all of us, wherever we are and regardless of which organisational development in primary care applies to our particular setting.

References

1 Comisión Americana Médico Social (2005) *Family Medicine at the Dawn of the Twenty First Century*. Mexico City: Conferencia Interamericano de Estudios de Seguridad Social, 5-6 September 2005.

2 Barnard K (2002) *Public Health and the Challenge of Implementing Primary Health Care: moving from an ideal world to ethical action*. Barcelona: WHO Office for Integrated Health Services.

3 Boaden N (1997) *Primary Care. Making connections*. Buckingham: Open University Press.

4 Starfield B (1998) *Primary Care. Balancing health needs, services, and technology*. New York: Oxford University Press.

5 WHO-UNICEF (1978) Primary Health Care. Report of the International Conference on Primary Health Care, Alma-Ata, USSR. Geneva: WHO Health for All Series No 1, 6–12 September.

6 WONCA Europe (2002a) *The European Definition of General Practice/Family Medicine*. Barcelona: WHO Office.

7 Boelan C, Haq C, Hunt V et al. (2002b) *Improving Health Systems: the contribution of family medicine*. Geneva: WONCA/WHO.

8 Dowell T, Neal R (2002) Vision and change in primary care: past, present and future. In: Tovey P (ed.) *Contemporary Primary Care. The challenge of change*, pp.9–25. Buckingham: Open University Press.

9 WHO (1998) *Primary Health Care 21: 'everybody's business'*. Geneva: WHO.

10 Sarriot E, Winch P, Ryan L et al. (2004) A methodological approach and framework for sustainability assessment in NGO-implemented primary health care programs. *International Journal of Health Planning and Management*. **19**: 23–41.

11 WHO (2001) *Guidelines on the Regional Primary Health Care Assessment*. Geneva: WHO.

12 Mullen F (1998) The 'Mona Lisa' of health policy: primary care at home and abroad. *Health Affairs*. **17**(2): 118–26.

13 Kark S (1981) *The Practice of Community-Oriented Primary Care*. New York: Appleton-Century-Crofts.

14 Gofin J (2001) The Community-Oriented Primary Care approach and Towards Unity for Health: unity of action and purpose. *Towards Unity for Health*. **1**: 9–10.

15 Bennet S, McPake B, Mills A (1007) The public/private mix debate in health care. In: Bennet S, McPake B, Mills A (eds) *Private Health Providers in Developing Countries*, pp.1–18. London: Zed Books.

16 Preston R (1996) *International Consultancy*. London: British Council.

17 Smith P (ed.) (2001) *The Primary Care Trust Handbook*. Oxford: Radcliffe Medical Press.

18 Meads G (ed.) (1996) *A Primary Care-led NHS: putting it into practice*. Edinburgh: Churchill Livingstone.

19 Niessen L, Grijseels E, Rutten F (2000) The evidence-based approach in health policy and health policy delivery. *Social Science and Medicine*. **51**: 859–69.

20 John P (1998) *Analysing Public Policy*. London: Continuum.

Index

Page numbers in *italic* refer to figures, tables and boxes.